Janet Balaskas is a childbirth educator, a ⟨…⟩ and ⟨…⟩ the Active Birth Movement, as well as being the mother of four children. She has campaigned for women to have the right to choose an Active birth and has helped effect change in maternity practices and midwifery education internationally. In 1987 she helped to organise the first International Conference on Home Birth, and is a founder of the International Home Birth Movement. She runs the Active Birth Centre in London.

New Active Birth

A concise guide to natural childbirth

JANET BALASKAS

Foreword by Sheila Kitzinger
Introduction by Michel Odent

Thorsons
An Imprint of HarperCollinsPublishers

Thorsons
An Imprint of HarperCollins*Publishers*
77–85 Fulham Palace Road,
Hammersmith, London W6 8JB

First published by Unwin Paperbacks in 1989.
Published by Thorsons 1991

10 9 8 7 6 5 4 3 2

British Library Cataloguing in Publication Data

Balaskas, Janet
    New active birth – Rev. ed,
    1. Natural childbirth. Preparation – Manuals
    I. Title   II. Balaskas, Janet. Active birth
    618.2'4

ISBN 0 7225 2566 4

Printed in Great Britain at the University Press, Cambridge

Photographs by Anthea Sieveking
Illustrations by Lucy Su and Laura McKechnie
Designed by Julia Lilauwala

Contents

Acknowledgements   *page*   *vi*
Preface *by Janet Balaskas*   *vii*
Foreword *by Sheila Kitzinger*   *xi*
Introduction *by Michel Odent*   *xii*

 1 What is an Active Birth?   1
 2 Your Body in Pregnancy   18
 3 Yoga-based Exercises for Pregnancy   30
 4 Breathing   79
 5 Massage   83
 6 Labour and Birth   89
 7 Water Birth   139
 8 After the Birth   149
 9 Postnatal Exercises   155
10 Active Birth at Home or in Hospital   161
11 A–Z Reference   191
    Active Birth Manifesto   201
    Recommended Reading   204
    Useful Addresses   205
    Reference List   207
    Index   209

Acknowledgements

First I would like to thank all of the mothers and their families whose experiences fill the pages of this book.

Thanks also to those who helped to produce it, especially Anthea Sieveking for the photographs, and the staff at Unwin Paperbacks for this new edition.

I am very grateful to my colleagues Lolly Stirk and Yvonne Moore for helping to establish the Active Birth Teachers Training Course; to Yehudi Gordon, Michel Odent and midwives everywhere for their pioneering work, as well as yoga teachers Mina Semyon, Mary Stuart, Lolly and John Stirk for their inspiration.

Profound thanks to Carole Eliott for her guidance and her husband Norman Stannard for his healing energy. Most of all I would like to thank my four children for helping me discover the great joy of giving birth and being a mother and my husband Keith Brainin for his loving support and encouragement.

For classes or teacher training in the Janet Balaskas method of preparation for Active Birth contact:
The Active Birth Movement
55 Dartmouth Park Road
London NW5 1SL

Preface

My first daughter, Nina, was born in 1970. I attended preparation classes and was hoping for a natural birth. I was active until strong labour began and then I lay passively in bed, semi-reclining, for the last three hours. Fortunately there were no complications and I managed, with enormous effort and the help of an unnecessary episiotomy, to give birth to her spontaneously.

I discovered active childbirth during the birth of my second daughter, Kim. During this pregnancy I had taken up yoga and enjoyed practising the yoga postures, finding some of them particularly beneficial as the pregnancy advanced. A study of the history of childbirth revealed how some of the yoga postures, especially squatting, had been used throughout the ages as birth positions. An anatomical study of the female pelvis clarified that these postures relaxed and 'opened' the pelvic canal and were ideal movements to adopt when trying to evacuate its contents.

Consequently, when it came to labour, I began by following the usual instructions given in antenatal classes and made myself comfortable in the semi-reclining position, focusing on some breathing techniques. Progress was slow and while the breathing techniques kept me calm and centred, they seemed to distract me from the labour. Eventually I decided to get up and try some of the positions I had practised during pregnancy. The change in progress was dramatic and it dawned on me, for the first time, that it is necessary for a woman to move and to be in harmony with gravity in order to help her body to open up in labour. I realised then, that squatting, and its variations, is the logical position for any woman to adopt while giving birth and is the most important position to practise during pregnancy. I resolved there and then to improve my squatting before my next labour.

During my son Iasonas's birth I kept active; walking, squatting and kneeling, and gave birth to him on all-fours. It was a marvellous experience. I had an entirely new sense of control and knew instinctively what to do. I was up within hours of the birth and felt none of the aches and pains I had for a week or two after my previous births, despite the fact that he was almost a 10lb baby. I was astonished how fit and well I felt after the birth, and suffered no exhaustion or depression in the following months.

Recently, number four was born, also at home. Theo weighed in at 11lbs and this time I had a portable water birth pool designed by my husband Keith, in our bedroom. Labour was intense and as soon as I reached 5cms dilation I entered the pool. The buoyancy of the water made it much easier for me to relax. I was encouraged to let myself go without any inhibitions, and I remember making a tremendous amount of noise and reaching full dilation very quickly.

Michel Odent, who was in attendance, suggested that I leave the pool for the actual birth. Given Theo's size, we decided that I needed the help of gravity to get him born, so I used the supported standing squat position. He was born in two contractions despite his size, miraculously without a tear. The medical establishment would certainly have considered me 'high risk'. I was 42, rhesus negative and had surgery on the uterus 3 years previously. These were the very reasons that I wanted to stay at home where conditions for a normal birth were optimal.

My own birth experiences are not unusual. Since 1978 I have been teaching yoga to pregnant women and more than 80 per cent of them have succeeded in giving birth naturally and actively to their babies. Most of them had no previous experience of yoga and their ages have ranged from 19 to 49. It has been a joy to observe how readily their bodies responded to the yoga. As their flexibility improved, their health and happiness increased. At the end of pregnancy most of them were in touch with their birthing and motherly instincts and could approach the birth with confidence. The experiences of these women have added to my personal conviction and won support from their midwives, doctors and obstetricians.

Many women enjoy the benefits of yoga so much that they are back in the mother and baby exercise sessions two to three weeks after birth. This is so, not only in the case of the mother who has a normal, problem-free birth, but also for those who have needed the help of forceps or Caesarean section.

Over the years I have seen that active labour and the adoption of natural, upright or crouching birth positions is the safest, most enjoyable, most economical and sensible way for the majority of women to give birth. There is no disruption of the normal physiology of labour, no interference with the hormonal balance, postnatal depression is rare and problems with breastfeeding and mothering are less likely.

The majority of labours – managed well – should be uncomplicated. No special equipment is needed and the birth can take place in the simplest environment or in the most sophisticated hospital delivery room.

Active Birth is natural and instinctive. Left to her own devices it is the way a woman will behave during labour. In preparing a woman for an active birth, my aim is to help her get in touch with her own birth-giving instinct.

Giving birth is essentially a natural bodily function, which occurs quite spontaneously and involuntarily at the end of pregnancy. It is part of a continuous evolution which begins with love-making and conception and ends in the growing independence of the child from his mother, during the first few years of life. The whole process of conceiving a baby, being pregnant, giving birth and mothering is part of the sexual and spiritual life of a woman, and is basically rooted in the natural and undisturbed unfolding of a series of physiological events.

The best way in which a woman, entering into motherhood, can prepare herself is from her own body.

The yoga exercises I recommend are not unnatural movements imposed upon the body. On the contrary, they are instinctive and simple movements we could all make with ease. It is a kind of physical 'remembering' rather than a system of exercise. In fact, many of the exercises in this book came from my observations of the movements made by my children when they were very young. By watching them, I realised how stiff, as adults, we have become; how we have lost contact with the range of movement nature intended us to have. A toddler will squat with ease for a long time, feet flat on the ground, back straight and rising up from this position when he learns to walk.

It is well known that the more civilised we become the more we forget our natural habits. Today we are able to ensure a reliable medical back-up for all women in the event of complications and the mortality rate has improved by the life-saving techniques of modern obstetrics. However, I have seen all too often in my practice, how the widespread use of routine obstetric technology, inappropriately applied to normal labour, disturbs the natural birth process and causes many of the problems it was designed to prevent. In some hospitals, birth has become an abdominal or vaginal extraction conducted on a conveyor belt. The result is that most women are completely out of touch with their own instinctive ability to give birth, and midwives are losing their intuitive skills as they depend more on technology. Many women have never seen a birth or even held a baby by the time they enter motherhood. The natural skills of giving birth and mothering are no longer handed down from woman to woman, generation to generation.

We can regain a link with our primitive female heritage by re-educating our bodies in the habits, movements and postures which are instinctive to the child-bearing woman. In pregnancy the whole tendency of the body is towards health and vitality and it is a unique opportunity for a woman to work on herself.

The main concern of this book is with normal birth and the common variations from the norm, which can usually be dealt with without obstetric intervention. Women who have prepared in this way and then found themselves faced with an unexpected complication or have needed the help of pain-relieving drugs, often find ways of successfully combining Active Birth with obstetric procedures.

I hope that this book will help to bring to light the simple common sense of childbirth which has somehow been obscured in the advance of modern obstetrics, and will help women to rediscover their own inner resources for giving birth to their babies.

THE ACTIVE BIRTH MOVEMENT

In the late 1970s a group of women in North London, recognising the benefits of Active Birth, attempted to give birth in upright positions in a local hospital.

Some of them met with success and were positively encouraged by obstetrician Yehudi Gordon and his staff to do so, while others encountered stubborn opposition. Conflict arose within the labour ward which resulted in a 'ban' being placed on Active Birth. Some mothers whose births were imminent, were extremely distressed and rang me to express their feelings. I felt responsible for introducing them to the concept. It seemed completely inappropriate for them to have to fight for the right to give birth instinctively, during their labours.

Consequently the Active Birth Movement was founded in April 1982 and the Active Birth Manifesto was written (see Chapter 11).

The occasion was marked by a demonstration on Sunday, 11 April which we called the Birthrights Rally. Originally, we intended to hold a 'squat-in' in the hospital foyer, but within a mere three weeks so many people were offering their support, that we ended up on Hampstead Heath with a crowd of 6,000. The rally was a protest against hospitals which denied women the right and freedom to move about in labour and to give birth in upright, squatting or kneeling positions, despite mounting evidence as to the advantages.

Michel Odent, whose work in France was featured in the same year on BBC2, was in London and came to speak at the rally along with Sheila Kitzinger, the newsreader Anna Ford, and other friends of Active Birth. The occasion was memorable and there was a change of attitude at the hospital which has been able to accommodate women wanting Active Births ever since. Thankfully, the Active Birth Movement has not needed to stage another demonstration as hospitals throughout London and further afield have gradually been adjusting to the climate of change. Although there is still a long way to go, the principles of Active Birth are being put into practice more widely, as our knowledge of the normal physiology of the birth process increases.

Our main function since then has been educational, providing conferences, lectures, workshops for parents and professionals, as well as training facilities for Active Birth teachers. We also provide a free advisory service from our London centre (see Useful Addresses).

The use of upright postures and mobility in labour are not unique to our part of the world and change has been happening simultaneously in many countries over the last decade. The Active Birth Movement is now international and has branches all over the world, many of whom have had great success in stimulating change. It is run entirely by women like myself, who have rediscovered childbirth through their own experiences. They are women who have chosen to get off the obstetric delivery table and to give birth instinctively. Consequently they pass on what they have learnt to others and through their work they are creating a new tradition of womanly wisdom, helping women everywhere to regain their autonomy as childbearers.

It is to them that I dedicate this book.

Foreword

Here is an important voice in childbirth. Janet Balaskas is speaking to those women who want to grow in self-awareness and to use their bodies actively in labour. In her childbirth classes Janet Balaskas stands for activity rather than passivity, for movement rather than immobilisation and a woman's right to choose whatever position she finds comfortable throughout labour and delivery.

The teaching in this book is revolutionary. Yet it is age-old. All over the world and throughout recorded history women have chosen upright positions to give birth and it is only we in the West who have had the extraordinary notion that a woman should lie on her back with her legs in the air to deliver a baby.

But to get women upright is to do much more than help them find a comfortable posture. It is to turn them from passive patients into active birth-givers. It is to challenge the whole obstetric view of birth in Western society. This is based on the assumption that childbirth is a medical event which should be conducted in an intensive care setting. The whole pregnancy is seen as a pathological condition terminated only by delivery. The modern high-tech obstetrician actively manages labour with all the technology of ultrasound, continuous electronic monitoring and oxytocin intravenous drip. Many obstetricians have never had the opportunity to see a truly natural birth. To turn the process of bringing new life into the world into one in which a woman becomes simply the body on the delivery table rather than an active birth-giver is a degradation of the mother's role in childbirth.

We are now beginning to discover the sometimes long-term destructive effects on the relationship between a mother and her baby and on the family, of treating women as if they were merely containers to be relieved of their contents and of concentrating attention on a bag of muscle and a birth canal, instead of relating to and caring for the person of whom the uterus and the vagina are a part.

'Bonding' is a fashionable term today. In many hospitals special time is devoted for bonding and there must be few midwives and obstetricians who would not claim that they consider bonding important. But everything that happens after delivery is the outcome of what has gone before. Bonding is either spontaneous and easy, or made virtually impossible by the atmosphere at delivery and by the care a woman is given as a *person*, not merely a 'para 1', an elderly primigravida, a maternal pelvis, a contracting uterus or a dilating cervix.

The way we give birth is important to all of us because it has a great deal to do with the kind of society we want to live in, the significance of the coming to birth of a new person and a new family.

When we hand over responsibility for choosing between alternatives on the basis of what we believe to be right, we hand over responsibility for the quality of the society we, and our children, must live in.   Sheila Kitzinger

Introduction

The concept of 'active birth' is a milestone in the history of childbirth. Bringing together these two simple words is by itself a work of genius: 'active birth' covers a huge scale of meanings, at different complementary levels.

The first level might be described as muscular. When you just have a glimpse of some pictures of 'active births' you notice that at the end of the labour, when the baby is coming, many mothers are vertical, hanging on to someone or something, or leaning forward on something, or in a supported squatting position, or kneeling . . .

At the second level you penetrate more deeply into the physiological process of childbirth. Childbirth is first a brain process. When a woman is giving birth by herself, the active part of her brain is the primitive part. It is this part which we have in common with all the mammals, the part which secretes the necessary hormones. A woman gives birth actively when she can secrete her own hormones, or, in other words, when she does not need synthetic hormones from a drip, or any other kind of medical intervention. The activity of the primitive part of the brain implies a reduction of inhibitions coming from the 'new' brain, the neocortex. The factors which can disturb this brain process, this change of conscious level, are not easily eliminated in the context of modern obstetric units: privacy, semi-darkness, silence, and, at the same time, the proximity of an experienced person.

At the third level 'active birth' refers to the attitude that society as a whole has towards childbirth. In our society childbirth is completely under the control and under the responsibility of medical institutions. Pregnant and labouring women are called 'patients'. Medical institutions include modern midwifery. Modern midwives, trained in obstetric units, are not any longer mothers helping other mothers. When a newborn baby is not healthy, the medical institution is considered as responsible. The concept of 'active birth' has been introduced by women who want to take back the control and the responsibility of childbirth. They consider the medical institution as a resource to use in precise circumstances. What a provocative challenge at a time when the negative side effects of obstetrics are better and better known!

The day when Janet introduced the phrase 'active birth' is possibly the most important one in the history of childbirth in Europe . . . since the day when the French doctor Mauriceau took control of this event and placed the labouring woman on her back.

Michel Odent

1 | What is an Active Birth?

During the rapid development of modern obstetrics in the last three hundred years, women have lost touch with their power as birth-givers. We have almost forgotten how a natural physiological birth unfolds.

An Active Birth is nothing new. It is simply a convenient way of describing normal labour and birth and the way that a woman behaves when she is following her own instincts and the physiological logic of her body. It is a way of saying that she herself is in control of her body while giving birth, rather than the passive recipient of an 'actively managed' birth on the part of her attendants.

By deciding to have an Active Birth you will be reclaiming your fundamental power as a birth-giver, a mother and also as a woman. You will also be giving your baby the best possible start in life and a safe transition from the womb to the world. Should an unusual difficulty or complication arise, you will be free to make use of the safety net of modern obstetric care, knowing that you have done your very best and also knowing that this is your choice and that the intervention was really necessary. In this way, even the most difficult birth can be a positive experience.

Preparing for an Active Birth during pregnancy will lessen the likelihood of complications arising. It will also ensure that you approach the birth of your baby in optimal health, which will enhance and hasten your recovery, whatever happens.

If you give birth actively you will want to move around freely during the early part, or first stage, of labour, choosing comfortable upright positions such as standing, walking, sitting, kneeling or squatting. In between contractions you will find ways to rest in these positions, comfortably supported by pillows. As you approach the expulsive or second stage during which your child will be born, you will continue to use the upright positions which are most comfortable or practical. At the end, for the actual birth, you will use a natural expulsive position (usually supported) like squatting or kneeling.

An Active Birth is instinctive. It involves you giving birth quite naturally and spontaneously through your own will and determination, having the complete freedom to use your body as you choose and to follow its urges. Active Birth is an attitude of mind. It involves acceptance and trust in the natural function and involuntary nature of the birth process, as well as an attitude or appropriate positioning of your body. It is not merely a vaginal extraction or delivery in which the attendants are in control and you are a passive patient. It is more comfortable, safer and more efficient than a passive 'confinement'. This is supported by the many scientific studies comparing women who are active in labour with those in a passive recumbent position (see page 207).

Some women, left to themselves, will instinctively know what to do in labour, but most of us, having no example to follow, need to be made aware of the possibilities of using various upright positions in order to discover our instincts. This can easily be done by practising the birth positions and movements which are most appropriate and comfortable during your pregnancy. The yoga-based exercises in this book will lead you towards your own instincts for labour and birth, while cultivating the right and natural body habits for a healthy pregnancy.

The Question of Birth Positions

A growing number of women, midwives, nurses, obstetricians and childbirth educators are questioning positions that characterise modern labour and birth practices, and the passive, patient-orientated role demanded of women in contemporary maternity care. The specific practice that is being criticised is the almost exclusive use of lying down (recumbent) positions for childbirth known as supine, dorsal or lithotomy positions. There is more than sufficient evidence that upright birth positions, i.e. kneeling, sitting, standing and squatting, are more advantageous to both mother and child.

Position and movement in labour is an area of fundamental importance which has been, in the past, almost completely neglected by birth attendants in the management of labour, and therefore also prenatal teachers in the preparation of women in birth. The choice of position determines the training of midwives and doctors. It also determines their approach and the kind of environment in which women labour and give birth. It can also determine the successful outcome of the birth and the quality of the experience for both mother and baby.

Modern Western Practice

Obstetric practice in the modern world is usually regarded as a medical, if not surgical, procedure. Until recently, the normal practice in most hospitals has been (and often still is) to place you, when you are in labour, in bed on your back; at best propped up by pillows into a semi-reclining position, where monitors, drips or anaesthetic can be conveniently applied. Later, just before the time of actual birth, you may be transferred to a delivery room and placed on an obstetric table where a forceps delivery, vacuum extraction, episiotomy or

Caesarian section can be performed, or, at best, your baby can be most conveniently 'delivered' by your attendants,

In many hospitals the choice of birth positions is already predetermined by the approach to maternity care and the routine hospital practices. Usually, the training of midwives and doctors takes the recumbent position for granted in specific obstetric practices, such as:

- The continuous assessment of foetal heart tones, uterine and other vital signs during labour and the use of electronic heart monitors which were designed for use in the recumbent position. Paradoxically, these often cause the foetal distress they are meant to detect by the imposition of the supine position for their use (1).
- Midwives are usually trained to do periodic vaginal examinations with the mother lying on her back. Where birth is active there is less need for vaginal examinations, as the progress of labour can usually be assessed by the mother's behaviour. If an internal examination is considered to be necessary, it can usually be done conveniently enough with the mother remaining upright.
- The use of sedatives, oxytocin drugs, analgesics and anaesthesia during labour and delivery. If the mother is not lying down in the first place she is less likely to need pain relief or induction.
- The use of forceps and/or episiotomy for delivery, or the need for the midwife to routinely 'control' the delivery or 'guard' the perineum. All these practices are not usually needed in an Active Birth.

When such practices are routinely used, labour and birth are seen from the outset as a potentially pathological situation in which attendants and their attendant technology are in control, rather than the woman herself, her instincts and her biological body.

No one will deny the enormous advantages of the safety net of modern obstetrics when problems occur which may threaten the life of mother or baby, or both. However, the vast majority of labours have the potential to be uncomplicated, and it is clear that common sense in the management of labour has been completely obscured by the routine application of interventive obstetrics to normal labour, resulting in a great increase in the number of forceps deliveries and Caesarean sections.

In many countries in the developed world the majority of babies born in hospital are delivered by forceps, or induced, or both, and the Caesarean rate may be as high as 30 per cent. In the USA, approximately one in four births (25 per cent) result in a Caesarean which reflects a 400 per cent increase in the last 20 years (2). In some hospitals, as many as one in three births are Caesarean, and in some large teaching hospitals the figure is closer to 60 per cent.

Amongst other reasons, the rigid insistence on making women in labour lie on their backs contributes largely to these figures. It seems that a vicious circle arises as soon as we begin to intervene in the natural process – the possibility of complication increases, the need for intervention and for pain-relieving drugs becomes more prevalent. When a labouring woman is immobilised and forced to lie on her back, the natural process is fundamentally disturbed and the likelihood of problems occurring increases.

What is wrong with obstetrically managed birth?

Giving birth can, and usually does involve hours of intense labour and a great deal of pain, effort and endurance on your part. Naturally the prospect is quite awesome and you will probably approach the birth of your child with some fear and apprehension about what is to come.

To many women the prospect of a painless, effortless, managed birth might, at first, seem to be an attractive proposition. After all, you might ask, why suffer needlessly when medication and modern technology is readily available to make the birth easier, quicker and less painful?

Regretably, it is not as simple as all that. Every interventive obstetric technique has known side effects for mother and baby, while many subtle or long-term effects may not yet be apparent. When help is genuinely needed the benefits of the intervention may well outweigh the risks. However, routine use of obstetric management tends to complicate birth unnecessarily.

Doris Haire in her booklet, *The Cultural Warping of Childbirth* (3), has written an excellent report on obstetrics in the USA where high-tech birth is the norm and more deeply entrenched than in most places, and now provides a model for developing countries where traditional birth practices are disappearing.

Haire points out that the infant mortality rate in the USA is amongst the highest in the world. There is also a staggering incidence of neurological impairment amongst American children which, she feels, is attributable largely to the 'unphysiological practises which have become so much a part of American obstetric care'. She lists an abundance of scientific literature and research to substantiate her remarks (see Recommended Reading).

We have known since the 1960s that all obstetric medications given to the mother, whether they are used to quell nausea, to induce labour, to relieve pain or to anaesthetise, do cross the placenta and do alter the baby's environment in the uterus, entering the baby's circulatory system and hence the baby's brain within seconds or minutes. Contrary to what many women are told, this includes regional anaesthetics such as epidurals (4).

The baby's central nervous system forms and develops rapidly in the last part of pregnancy, during the birth itself and during infancy, and is susceptible to the effects of drugs given around the time of birth and after. We have only to recall the thalidomide tragedy to realise that the testing of the safety of these medications is often sorely inadequate. Of course, it is important also to bear in mind that babies vary in their vulnerability to the effects of these drugs and, in instances of real need, the judicious and minimal use of medication is usually successful. However, in antenatal clinics and hospitals, mothers are usually uninformed about the hazards or side effects involved in taking such medications and are deluded into assuming that there are no risks involved.

Let us take a look at some examples of the most widely used medications for labour and birth, and their more common side effects. I have deliberately omitted the more severe and rare complications but readers who are interested can look up the research references listed on page 207.

THE PROMISE OF PAIN RELIEF

Pethidine (Demerol in the USA)

This is a narcotic-like analgesic used to 'take the edge' off pain. Given usually as an intramuscular injection, some women find it makes labour more tolerable and others that it causes them to lose control. There are possible side effects to the mother, such as nausea or dizziness, and it will slow down the mother's breathing and respiration, hence reducing the baby's oxygen supply. Often Pethidine is mixed with sedatives to reduce nausea and these too will cause sleepiness and enter the baby's bloodstream.

It is now common knowledge that Pethidine can depress the baby's respiratory system and jeopardise the start of breathing after birth, resulting in the need to resuscitate the baby (5).

Traces sometimes remain in the baby's system after birth so that, in addition to adjusting to life outside the womb, the baby's system will have the added burden of detoxification (6). They can also depress the baby's sucking reflex and because they remain in the baby's system for several weeks they can affect the initiation of breastfeeding and mother-infant bonding (7).

Epidurals

This is known as a regional anaesthetic which is injected locally into the epidural space between two lumbar vertebrae in the lower spine. When it works effectively the result will be a blocking of pain impulses, bringing numbness from the waist through the lower body.

While the effects of the drugs used for epidurals on the baby are not the same as Pethidine, we know that they enter the baby's circulation and brain tissues within minutes (6). Their immediate and long-term effects on the neurological development of the baby are relatively unknown and direly under-researched, despite the widespread use of this form of pain relief, worldwide.

Side effects for the mother, such as severe headaches following the birth, can occasionally occur (these are caused by accidental scratching of the membrane surrounding the spinal cord by the injection needle), and a lowering of maternal blood pressure is common.

An epidural will certainly increase the need for obstetric intervention. Of course the mother will be immobile and reclining so contractions tend to be less efficient, and labour is often much longer and may need to be artifically stimulated with an oxytocic drip.

All these factors contribute to a lessening of the blood supply to and from the uterus, so foetal distress (lack of oxygen) is far more likely. Sometimes the pelvic muscles become limp and do not help the baby to rotate in the usual way (with the added disadvantage of being without the help of gravity).

An epidural can also inhibit the mother's ability to push her baby out spontaneously and, one way or another, the risk of a forceps delivery or a Caesarean section is increased.

When mothers give birth actively, with the help of a midwife, the forceps rate rarely rises above 5 per cent and drugs are only used in cases of unavoidable distress or to save a life. By contrast, in countries such as the USA, the incidence of forceps deliveries can be, according to Doris Haire, as high as 65 per cent in some hospitals. An unnecessary forceps delivery can be traumatic for both mother and child and can occasionally result in injury or damage to the baby (8).

Although, at times, the total freedom from pain offered by an epidural may be indispensable, it is important, for a successful outcome, to weigh this advantage against the attendant risks, which are considerable. Occasionally the price of a few hours of comfort can be a damaged baby and may very well be a complicated birth (9–12).

So, might it not be better in the long run to learn how to use your body to release, minimise and transform the pain of labour and to have access to a pool of warm water or a shower – an effective and totally harmless way to reduce pain? If an epidural is really needed, then its use can be minimal and, in this way, the attendant risks are reduced.

STIMULATING LABOUR

Induction
An induction may be used to initiate labour or to stimulate contractions once it has begun. It is usually done by introducing an intravenous drip of Syntocinon (Pitocin in USA), a powerful synthetic hormone, into a vein in the mother's arm.

Normally, when the uterus contracts, the blood vessels which carry blood to the placenta are temporarily constricted. In between contractions, blood is stored in the placenta to keep up a constant supply to the baby during contractions. When contractions are stimulated by Syntocinon they tend to be longer, stronger and closer together than in a normal labour. The periods of constriction are therefore longer than usual so that the overall oxygen supply to the baby is reduced and foetal distress is therefore more likely. Doris Haire writes in *Drugs in Labour and Birth*, 'The situation is somewhat analogous to holding an infant under water and allowing the infant to come to the surface to gasp for air but not to breathe.'

The incidence of postnatal jaundice in babies who have been induced is also thought to be higher (13–14).

In addition, strong contractions usually occur as soon as the drip begins to work so the gradual build-up in intensity of a normal labour is absent. This often means that the mother cannot cope with the pain of the stronger contractions and will need pain relief, so the baby will end up with the combined effect of painkillers and the drugs used for induction.

Of course, continuous foetal monitoring will probably be necessary with all these risks and so the snowball effect continues as one intervention necessitates another.

Studies have shown that there is no evidence of any natural advantage in routinely inducing births that are 'overdue' and a failed induction frequently ends up as a Caesarean section (15–18).

Would it not be better to reserve this option as a last resort and discover how to change position to stimulate contractions, or how to improve the birthing environment so that the mother can secrete her own natural hormones? Learning how to allow the normal physiology to unfold without disturbance is the most effective way to ensure that the mother will secrete her own hormones.

Birth Before Obstetrics

Historical studies show the prevalent use of vertical positions – kneeling, squatting, standing or sitting postures – with many variations and as many methods of support.

There is evidence going back thousands of years of the bodily positions taken in childbirth. The head of a silver pin from Luristan in Iran, first millenium BC, depicts a squatting mother. The remains of a clay statue of 5750 BC from a shrine at Çatal Hüyük, a Copper Age (Chalcolithic) city in Turkey, shows a goddess giving birth in the same position, as does an 8½ inch Aztec stone fertility figure from Mexico. A relic of the Mound Builders of eastern Arkansas, a pre-Columbian culture of unknown date, shows a woman squatting with her hands on her thighs. The Egyptian hieroglyph meaning 'to give birth' shows a mother squatting.

A relief from the temple of Kom Ombo, a town on the Nile in Upper Egypt, shows a woman giving birth in the kneeling position. Birth in the same position can be seen in a marble figure from Sparta, about 500 BC. In ancient China and Japan, women customarily gave birth in the kneeling position on a straw mat. All scenes, of course, depict only the final birth, but positions used during the rest of labour can also be traced.

In the Old Testament, Exodus, chapter I, verse 16 states:

When ye do the office of a midwife to the Hebrew women, and see them upon the stools . . .

A Corinthian vase depicts a woman in labour seated on a birthchair. An early Greek relief and a Roman marble bas-relief both show a woman giving birth on a stool supported by two assistants. The birthstool was also recommended for uncomplicated labours by Soranus in the early part of the second century AD and by many subsequent writers. It was described as, 'In a form like a barber's chair but with a crescent-shaped opening in the seat through which the child may fall.' The first birthstools may have been rocks or logs of wood, developing over time into complex, adjustable chairs with many varied devices.

There are also many examples of women giving birth without a stool using a variety of upright postures and always supported by one or more attendants while the midwife receives the baby.

From Birthchair to Bed to Delivery Table

In the Western world, the birthstool or chair remained indispensably part of the equipment of most midwives up to the middle of the eighteenth century. Each wealthy household had its own stool, whilst among the poor a stool was transported from house to house. The birthstools of royalty were carved and ornamented with jewels. Dutch, German and French sixteenth century drawings show the great use of birthstools, as do Chinese drawings of the same period. Even today, a birthchair is still used by some Egyptian women.

The first record of a woman lying down for birth describes Madame de Montespan, mistress of Louis XIV, who lay down in a recumbent position so that he could watch the birth from behind a curtain. Then in the mid seventeenth century in France, two brothers named Chamberlain invented the forceps. The best position for a forceps delivery is to have the woman lying down. This invention was jealously guarded by the Chamberlains who performed their deliveries shrouded by black drapes, but the obstetric fashion for ladies of quality to give birth in recumbent positions became firmly entrenched, and the physician took over from the midwife in the birth chamber. In the same century, François Mauriceau became the leading figure in French obstetrics. He scorned the use of the birthchair and advocated childbirth in bed, lying on the back. As forceps gained popularity, the birthchair lost favour and, by the end of the eighteenth century, little more was heard of it.

In the nineteenth century, Queen Victoria was the first woman in England to have chloroform while giving birth. Delivery under anaesthetic further established the lying down position on the back or on the side. Birth positions which lend themselves more easily to the convenience of the attendants who perform these procedures became the only choice, and the practice of confining a woman to bed for the major part of her labour and then on to an obstetric table for delivery, eventually spread throughout the West. This practice has become so widespread that the word 'confinement' is commonly used to describe the birth process.

The birthchair had given way to the bed and the delivery tables of the nineteenth and twentieth centuries. Women were flat on their backs, a position that made them passive and controllable, and although this offered a fine view to the attendant, it was in total defiance of the active forces of gravity and the joyous independence that comes from naturally and instinctively giving birth actively, on one's own two feet.

Ethnological Evidence

Primitive tribes have adopted various birth positions through the customs of their tribe but, more important, by their instinct. Some forty positions have been recorded, and their relative merits have been much disputed. Women of different tribes squat, kneel, stand, incline, sit or lie on the belly; so, too, do they vary their positions in various stages of labour and in difficult labours.

Dr G. J. Englemann, in his book *Labour Among Primitive Peoples* written in 1883, was one of the first to investigate the various positions assumed in labour or childbirth by early people, and he found that the four principal positions were squatting, kneeling (including the all fours and knee-chest positions), standing and semi-recumbent.

Ethnologists entirely confirm the evidence of the historians. Whatever the race or the tribe under observation – African, American, Asian and so on, the same upright positions always predominate with a great variety of means of support. Figures reveal that, for the most part, women throughout the world today still labour and deliver in some form of upright or crouching position, usually supported.

Recent studies

Over the last few decades, as disillusionment with the routine application of high-tech obstetrics has increased, researchers all over the world have begun to explore normal physiological birth. Documented evidence has been available for over fifty years as to the physiological advantages of labour in upright, crouching positions. Certain principles of physics apply to childbirth and these are denied or negated when a woman gives birth lying down. The facilitating influence of squatting positions was also radiographically confirmed in the 1930s. It was shown that the cross-sectional surface area of the birth canal may increase by as much as 30 per cent when a woman changes from lying down on her back to the squatting position (19). And it is some twenty years since Scott and Kerr demonstrated the disadvantages of having the weight of a pregnant uterus pressing down on the back. Lying supine, the weight of the contracting uterus reduces the placental blood flow by compressing the large artery of the heart (the descending aorta) and the large veins leading to the heart (inferior vena cava). This is a hard clinical fact which should not be ignored by anyone involved with childbirth (20).

Most recent studies have revealed the definite advantages to a woman when she is walking about assuming upright positions during labour. The few, and they are a very small minority, who have not found any measurable advantage all conclude that there is definitely no disadvantage to being active and using upright positions during labour.

The majority of studies have established a control group and an experimental group. This has usually required that the control group remain supine or in some recumbent position in bed and that the experimental group assume an upright posture, sitting, squatting, kneeling or walking about. But other studies, which seem more convincing, have used the women as their own controls, asking them to alternate every thirty minutes between two positions – horizontal and upright – during the first and second stages of labour. These alternative approaches to examining the effect of position during labour both reveal similar positive results in favour of active upright labour and deliveries.

During the 1970s many studies were carried out in various parts of the world. In 1977, a study in Birmingham Maternity Hospital compared a group of women who walked about during labour with a group that lay down horizontally throughout most of labour. The results showed that the duration of labour was significantly shorter, the need for analgesics far less and the incidence of foetal heart abnormalities markedly smaller in the ambulant group than in the recumbent group. Women walking about also experienced less pain with uterine contractions, and they felt more comfortable upright. They concluded convincingly that walking about during labour, especially early labour, should be encouraged (21).

In Latin America, Dr Roberto Caldeyro-Barcia organised a collaborative study involving two maternity hospitals. Vertical labour positions (sitting and standing) and horizontal positions (side lying and lying on the back) were studied. Their effects on the labour and on the condition of the baby were compared (22). In 1972 in America, Dr Isaac N. Mitie of Indiana compared women in the second stage of labour, half of whom were lying down and the other half in sitting positions (23). Dr Yuen Chou Lui headed a study of sixty women in labour in two hospitals, one in New York City and the other in Washington (24).

These are a few of the many studies giving positive evidence of the benefits of walking about and using upright labour and birth positions. Most studies confirmed that uterine contractions were stronger and more efficient in dilating the cervix. Even though these studies were carried out in birthing environments which could be improved, the results were already impressive when only the attitude to posture was changed.

Results of Modern Research

Most studies reported that when upright and moving about the following advantages ensued:

1   The intensity (strength) of uterine contractions was found to be greater.
2   Greater regularity and frequence of uterine contractions.
3   The dilation or opening of the cervix (the neck of the uterus) was more efficient.
4   More complete relaxation between contractions.
5   The pressure of the baby's head on the cervix during the resting phase between uterine contractions was consistently higher.

6   The first and second stages of labour were shorter (some comparative studies showed they were over 40 per cent shorter in the upright group).
7   Greater comfort, less stress and pain and so decreased requirement for analgesics.
8   Lower incidence of foetal distress in labour and improved condition of the newborn.
9   Women felt they were contributing something to their labour and felt relieved from the boredom and degradation of lying down connected to equipment.

Why is Active Birth Better?

What explains the fact that women have easier labours and births when they move about and assume upright positions?

Common sense and recent studies suggest that, in upright positions, these are the advantages to mother and baby:

1   The pull of gravity, i.e. the earth's downward gravitational force, assists uterine contractions and bearing down efforts. It is easier for any object to fall towards the earth's surface than to slide parallel to it (Newton's Law of Gravity), so that it is mechanically more advantageous to expel an unborn baby towards the earth than to expel it along the horizon. In upright positions such as standing, squatting or kneeling, the mother's body is in harmony with the downward force of gravity. When she lies down her involuntary efforts to expel the baby spontaneously are inhibited, increasing the need for strenuous effort to push the baby 'uphill' or the need for a forceps extraction. Dr Peter Dunn, Consultant Senior Lecturer in Child Health at Southmead Hospital in Bristol, writing on the recumbent position for labour in *The Lancet* in 1976, noted, 'No animal species adopts such a disadvantageous posture during such an important and critical event' (25).
2   The drive angle of the uterus, i.e. the angle between the long axis of the unborn baby's spinal column and that of the mother's spinal column, is less when upright, so demanding less effort from the uterus. The uterus tilts forward when it contracts. In an upright position where the mother can lean forward, she is assisting her uterus to work with least resistance whereas, if she is lying down or leaning back, the uterus has to work harder against the downward force of gravity (see page 98). A muscle working against gravity tends to tire and ache more easily so leaning forward is an efficient way to reduce pain and the need for analgesics.
3   In between contractions, the increased pressure of the abdominal wall, the diaphragm and the baby's head all in turn increase the pressure on the cervix during the resting phase.
4   The entrance of the baby's head, or presenting part, to the inlet of the mother's pelvis is easier and the head's direct application to the mother's cervix is assisted, because the pelvic inlet points forward and the outlet

faces downward, producing a convenient angle of descent. With each contraction of the uterus the unborn baby has a tendency to sink towards the mother's cervix.

5   There is improved placental circulation giving better oxygen supply to the foetus. Lying down on one's back is the one position that causes compression of the major abdominal blood vessels along the spinal column. Compression of the large artery of the heart (descending aorta) can cause foetal distress by hindering blood circulation around the uterus and the placenta. Compression of the large veins leading to the heart (inferior vena cava) blocks the returning blood flow, contributing to hypotension and the possibility of maternal haemorrhage.

6   There is less pressure on the pelvic nerves stemming from the lower part of the spine and sacrum, and less resistance to the uterine effort, therefore there is less pain.

7   During pregnancy the flexibility of the pelvic joints is increased by hormones that soften the ligaments that hold them together. In upright positions, the pelvic joints are free to expand, move and adjust to the shape of the descending head of the baby during labour and birth. When the sacrum is free to move, the pelvic outlet can widen by as much as 30 per cent more (i.e. in the squatting position) than when the mother's weight is resting directly on it and preventing any movement (i.e. semi-reclining). The sacro-coccygeal joint, i.e. the joint between the sacrum and the coccyx or tailbone, also softens and is designed to swivel backwards to widen the outlet of the pelvis as the baby emerges. Of course, this is impossible if the mother is sitting on her coccyx (i.e. semi-sitting position).

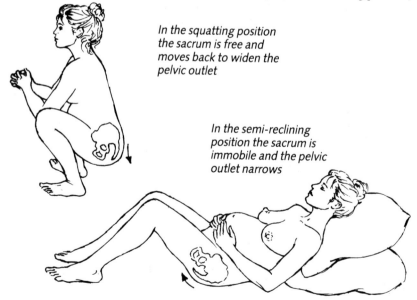

In the squatting position the sacrum is free and moves back to widen the pelvic outlet

In the semi-reclining position the sacrum is immobile and the pelvic outlet narrows

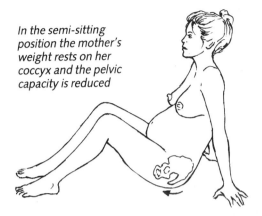

In the semi-sitting position the mother's weight rests on her coccyx and the pelvic capacity is reduced

8   When the mother is upright there is less direct pressure on the baby's neck vertebrae as the head passes under the pubic arch and the neck extends backwards during the second stage (see diagram on page 23). Although no studies have yet been done, it is easy to observe how actively-born babies have better head control immediately after birth. This facilitates the 'rooting reflex' for breastfeeding and also enhances motor development after birth.

9   Upright positions facilitate the successful and spontaneous separation of the placenta and reduce the need for controlled cord traction and the risk of post-partum infection or haemorrhage (26).

10   There is less likelihood of infection as fluids can drain more easily when the mother is upright and 'pooling' does not occur.

11   In an upright position, the perineal tissues can expand evenly and pull back around the baby's head, emerging at birth, and the risk of tearing is reduced. In the semi-reclining or semi-sitting position the baby's head descends forward directly onto the perineum which is immobilised and cannot expand. This situation is worsened if the mother is in the lithotomy position with her legs in stirrups. This separates the legs to a much great extent than usual and actually stretches the perineal tissues, increasing the need for episiotomy. In an active birth episiotomy is rarely necessary and is usually only done in an emergency.

Implications

Based on research findings, various up-to-date studies and ancestral instinct, it is foreseeable that widespread changes with respect to labour and birth positions are inevitable in the management of labour and in the preparation of women for childbirth (27–30).

As changes in position help to increase the strength and effectiveness of contractions, allowing a woman to be up and to walk about in early labour, especially if there are no complications, seems rational and good practice. A woman's own instincts dictate to her that she should move around. Standing, walking about and assuming various sitting, kneeling and squatting positions, with any suitable means of support, causes the uterus to exert more pressure on the foetus and in turn on the cervix. Women should be guided more by their own feelings, comfort and need rather than by hospital convenience and obstetric fashion. Freedom of one's body is necessary to find those positions which traditionally have been used to facilitate labour and delivery; positions which will assist one to attain maximum comfort, relaxation, ease and control.

There is an infinite range of possible positions and no constant chronological order. It is the need to search for the most effective, efficient and comfortable positions that is common. The common need amongst women instinctively to keep changing positions will one day have to be universally recognised. This involves a different attitude to the management of labour, to maternity care generally and to antenatal preparation.

A prospective mother needs not only knowledge of pregnancy, labour and delivery and the growth and development of babies, but also adequate physical preparation concerning the effects of varying upright positions and the cultivation of ease and comfort in them, so that she can actively and effectively help herself during labour. The emphasis during pregnancy will need to be on developing trust and confidence in her own body and on learning to discover her instinctive potential for childbirth and mothering. Her emotional and physical readiness for birth and her self-empowerment in pregnancy will become as important as good medical care in the antenatal clinic.

Squatting

Freedom to change position is more important than a single, optimal or best position during labour. It is unlikely that any woman would elect to remain in one position throughout labour. However, squatting is closest to nature's laws and is known as the physiological position. A position is physiologically effective:
- when there is no compression on the vena cava and the aorta
- when the pelvis becomes fully mobilised

Supported squatting seems to be especially efficient at the end of the second stage when the baby is being born. The squatting position produces:
- maximum pressure inside the pelvis
- minimal muscular effort
- optimal relaxation of the perineum
- optimal foetal oxygenation
- a perfect angle of descent in relation to gravity

A supported squat is essential in a breech delivery as it reduces delay between delivery of the umbilicus and the head.

Another useful position is the all fours position. The presenting part rotates inside the pelvis more easily when a woman is on all fours. This position can be especially useful if the baby is lying posterior or the birth is very fast.

None of the women in all the recent studies were prenatally prepared to gain ease and comfort in the squatting, kneeling, crouching and all fours position. How much better would the upright groups of women have fared if they had the additional benefit of physical preparation. (A controlled study of this kind has not yet been done.)

Ideal Maternity in Pithiviers, France

Michel Odent and his staff have provided a setting for women to be active in labour at the maternity unit in the general hospital in Pithiviers in France. Here, for two decades, women in labour have had the freedom to follow their instincts in walking about and finding positions that are suitable and comfortable. He and his midwives, together with expectant mothers, have discovered many means of physical support during labour and delivery which have proved, over the years, to be a tremendous advantage in easing labour and especially delivery. They do not use continuous foetal monitoring, Pethidine, epidurals or forceps. Few episiotomies are given and induction is very rare. Their concept of obstetrics, to try not to disturb the normal physiology, is very different from conventional practice aimed at control. Also the physical and the human environment is very different – the birthing room has a home-like rather than a hospital atmosphere.

In this unit there are about 1,000 deliveries a year. Professional care is the responsibility of Dr Odent and six midwives. The midwives work in pairs for forty-eight hours at a time followed by four days off. Each woman is given her own room throughout her stay and there are few rules. As labour advances, she walks to the birth room which has a low-level platform with many cushions, and a wooden squatting stool. There she is encouraged to remain active and change her position as many times as she wishes.

Most women prefer to walk about, sit on the birthstool, kneel on all fours, squat and lean on their husband or the midwifes for physical support. Water is regarded as important and women, if they like, may take a warm bath or relax in a small pool which is available. No drugs are used, the membranes are not artificially ruptured. Most women adopt an upright position for delivery, usually a supported squat; others give birth on the birthstool or on the low double bed and some give birth in water. With the appropriate supported squat and the minimum disturbance of the expulsive reflex, there are no unnecessary perineal tears and episiotomies are rare.

After the birth, the baby's bath and the delivery of the placenta, the mother walks with her husband and her newborn back to her own room. Of the 1,000 births that took place in Pithiviers in 1981, only eight babies needed intensive care.

Here is a maternity-care setting close to ideal. It has the safety of hospital delivery as well as the relaxed atmosphere of a comfortable and homely birth room. It is free of the frustrating regulations or limitations of routine hospital practices and is based on understanding of the instinctive behaviour of a woman in labour and her needs. They have a positive approach to an active, physiological birth with a natural outcome. The attendants are well-known to the mother and are constantly available during labour and delivery. Fathers participate and give their support. Women are given the freedom to move and adopt any position they find comfortable and the minimum use of drugs and interventions during labour are needed.

If the majority of women at Pithiviers can experience Active Birth safely and naturally in such a unit, why not elsewhere?

RESULTS OF 898 BIRTHS AT PITHIVIERS IN 1980

		% per thousand
* Perinatal deaths	8	10
Caesareans	44	5.0
Episiotomies	71	8.0
Vacuum extractions	57	6.3
Manual removal of placenta	10	1.1
Total previous Caesareans	26	2.9
Vaginal deliveries after previous Caesareans	18	2.0
** Transfers to pediatric unit	15	1.7
Forceps	0	

* All deaths after 6 months gestation
**Severe jaundice, malformations and premature

Since the time of writing, Michel Odent is no longer living in France and is based in London where his work continues with women giving birth at home. There are now many similar units and the results of their work reflect the same striking contrast to hospitals where obstetric management is still routine.

Your Responsibility

If the freedom to move and adopt upright positions makes sense to you and you want to give birth actively but do not have access to a maternity unit like Pithiviers, how can you go about it? You will have to make the possibility of an Active Birth your own responsibility; you will have to prepare your body to cultivate ease and comfort in upright positions as well as find a midwife, doctor or obstetrician (whether you wish to give birth at home or in hospital) who will support you in giving birth actively without the conventional intervention.

In parts of Britain, Europe, North and South America, Australia, New Zealand and elsewhere, increasing numbers of women, doctors, midwives and antenatal teachers are teaching and putting Active Birth into practice. Small groups are springing up everywhere spreading their message by word of mouth. (See page ix for The Active Birth Movement.) The women who form these groups have the proof of experiencing an active birth without drugs, without episiotomies and without tears. They prepare themselves to give birth actively by finding antenatal teachers who encourage them in this and they find doctors and midwives, maternity units and staff, who are prepared and willing to assist them to move about and use upright positions. If you want to give birth actively it will be helpful if you make contact with one of these consumer groups who help themselves to give birth actively and naturally. (See page 205 for useful names and addresses.) If this is not possible, you will have to persuade your doctor or midwife or whoever to enable you to follow these suggestions. The support of your partner can be very helpful. If he is willing to join you in preparing for an Active Birth, his presence at the birth can contribute greatly to a successful outcome.

SUGGESTIONS FOR LABOUR

During the first stage of labour while the cervix is dilating it is usually best to be upright and walking about, or kneeling during the contractions and resting in between them.

During the second stage, standing or kneeling with the upper body leaning well forward during contractions helps to complete the rotation of the head. At the end of the second stage, supported squatting seems to be the most effective and comfortable position during contractions. Squatting, especially supported, gives the greatest increase of pressure in the pelvic cavity with minimal muscular effort and optimal relaxation.

Some women prefer to kneel on all fours for delivery, particularly if the second stage is very quick.

It is wise to make a point of meeting your midwife or doctor, or the midwife in charge of the labour ward, to discuss these ideas early in pregnancy if possible. As you read this book it will be helpful to list the issues that are important to you so that you can go through them together, and then attach a copy to your notes for easy reference by the midwife who attends you in labour. When labour starts it may help to request a midwife who is enthusiastic about natural, active birth and who has had previous experience in the use of upright postures.

2 | Your Body in Pregnancy

The Pelvic Organs

Your uterus lies deep inside your abdominal cavity, between the bladder in front and the rectum behind. These are known as the pelvic organs. Your abdominal cavity extends from your diaphragm, beneath your lungs, to the muscles of the floor of your pelvis.

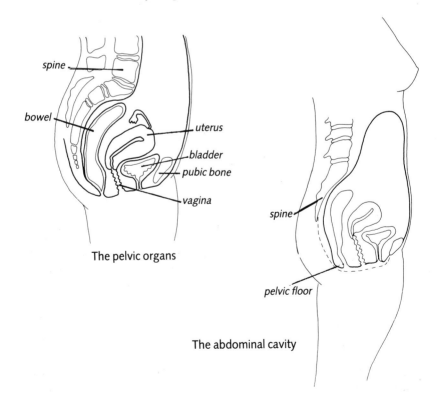

The pelvic organs

The abdominal cavity

Before pregnancy your uterus is a small, hollow muscular organ, shaped like an inverted pear, measuring roughly 3ins. × 2ins. × 1in. Extending to each side from the top part, or *fundus*, are two narrow canals, the Fallopian tubes, and these end in finger-like projections called *fimbria* which surround your ovaries on either side and draw up the ripe *ovum* after you ovulate. The lower part or mouth of the uterus is called the cervix which projects into the vagina and will open up during labour to allow your child to be born. During pregnancy your cervix is closed and the narrow opening is sealed with a mucous plug. The cervix is about 1½ inches long.

The uterus is the principal organ involved in pregnancy and childbirth. Your child is conceived in one of its Fallopian tubes, implanted within its cavity and, at the appropriate time, is expelled by it through your vagina into the outside world.

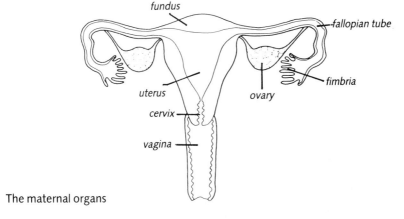

The maternal organs

During the forty weeks of pregnancy, your uterus increases in size to about 12ins. × 9ins. × 9ins. Its weight increases from 100 grams to 1,000 grams at full term and the amount of fluid it contains grows from a quarter of a teaspoon to approximately 1½ pints.

During the first sixteen weeks of pregnancy, the expansion of your uterus is caused almost entirely by the growth of its tissues owing to hormonal stimulation. The uterus becomes a thick-walled organ, circular in shape and is protected and cradled by the bones of your pelvis. Around this time you will begin to feel the 'quickening' movements of your child within the womb.

From the twentieth week, growth almost ceases and the uterus then expands because the muscle fibres are stretched by the growing child. At the very end of pregnancy, the lower segment of the uterus stretches most which is why a low-lying placenta will tend to rise as the uterine walls lengthen at the base. The walls of the uterus become thinner and in the latter half of the pregnancy you can feel your child's body quite easily from outside. Your uterus becomes more oval in shape and moves up into your abdomen as your child grows.

As it enlarges, its position changes. At 12 weeks the fundus is just above your pelvic inlet. At 16 weeks, its upper end is nearly halfway to your navel, which it reaches at the eighteenth week. At 36 weeks, the top part of your uterus is lying just below your diaphragm, at the level of the lower end of your breastbone. During the last few weeks it drops a little lower as your baby settles into position for birth.

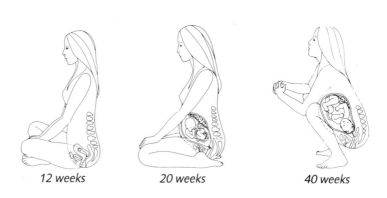

12 weeks   *20 weeks*   *40 weeks*

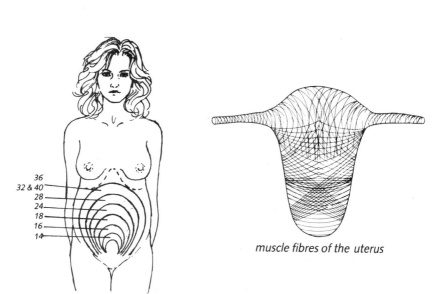

varying levels of the uterus

muscle fibres of the uterus

Your uterus is a hollow muscular organ which consists of a network of muscle fibres and bundles running in all directions, longitudinal, oblique and circular.

During pregnancy your baby lies within the uterus connected from his navel by the umbilical cord to the placenta which is attached to the wall of your uterus and draws nourishment for your child from your bloodstream and, simultaneously, passes waste products back to you. The placenta usually implants in the upper segment of the uterus towards the back but variations within the norm sometimes occur. The umbilical cord is made up of three intertwined blood vessels, two veins carrying oxygenated blood from the placenta back to the baby and one artery which carries de-oxygenated blood from the baby to the placenta.

Your baby has an independent blood circulation system which flows all round the body through the umbilical cord to the placenta and back again. After the birth, when your baby is breathing independently, the placenta is no longer needed and will separate from the wall of the uterus and pass through the cervix. Your baby's placenta is about one-third of the size of your baby and is lined by the membranes. It looks like a large piece of liver. If it is examined and spread out one can see that it is a network of blood vessels, rather like the roots of a tree.

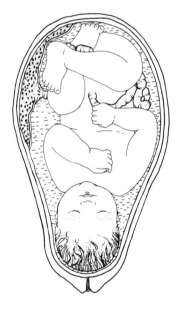

Baby at term in the womb surrounded by waters and membranes with cord and placenta

A bag of membranes surrounds your baby, the placenta and cord and also contains approximately 1½ pints of amniotic fluid – the waters within which your baby lies. These waters protect your baby from shock or infection and are constantly being replenished by your body.

At full term, at the end of pregnancy, the main function of your uterus is to evacuate its contents. During labour the uterus will contract at regular intervals and gradually open up at its base (the cervix) to allow your baby to pass through. Once it has opened, it will contract powerfully to expel your baby and the placenta, the bag of membranes and all its contents. (Placenta and membranes are called the 'after birth'.) In the hours and weeks after the birth, your uterus will continue to contract rhythmically, stimulated by hormones. Your baby sucking on the breast will stimulate the release of these contracting hormones. The uterus will gradually shrink back to its original shape and size and will expel all the blood-rich lining which was used to nourish your baby. By the end of the sixth week after birth, your uterus will be back to normal and will have completed its task.

The Pelvic Bones

Your pelvis is the part of your body most directly involved with giving birth. It is the bony passage through which your baby will pass as it is born. During pregnancy your body produces hormones which soften the joints in order to increase their flexibility and assist the birth of your child. By regularly practising the exercises recommended in the next chapter, you can make the most of this natural flexibility and be at your physical best for giving birth.

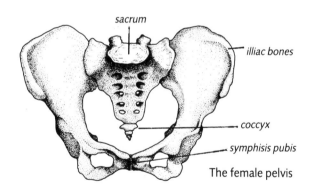

The female pelvis

TRY THIS:

a Kneel on the floor and explore your pelvis from the outside. Place your hands on your hips and find the illiac crests – two bony points at your sides – and follow their curved rim with your thumbs round to the back. Feel your pubic bone in front, your sacrum and coccyx at the back.
b Sit on your hands and feel your two buttock bones.

c Kneel, then lift up one foot so that you are half-kneeling and half-squatting. Explore your pubic arch. Feel its curve extending from your buttock bones under your pubic bone. Your baby's head will pass under this arch as it is born.

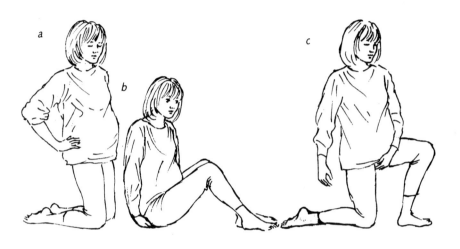

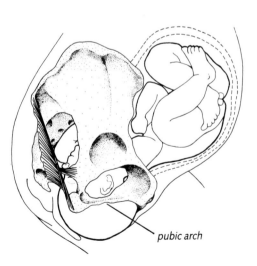

pubic arch

Your pelvis is shaped internally like a curved funnel – exactly the right shape to accommodate your baby's head as it passes through during labour. From above you can see the pelvic inlet in which your baby's head will engage, ready to be born; and from underneath the outlet through which it passes at birth.

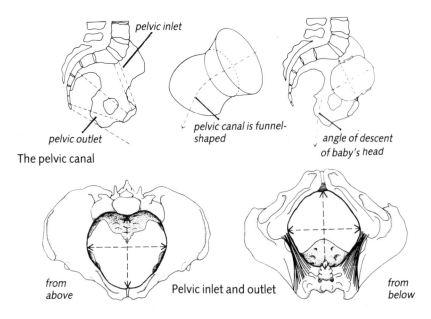

pelvic inlet

pelvic outlet

The pelvic canal

pelvic canal is funnel-shaped

angle of descent of baby's head

from above   Pelvic inlet and outlet   *from below*

Your pelvis has 4 major joints.

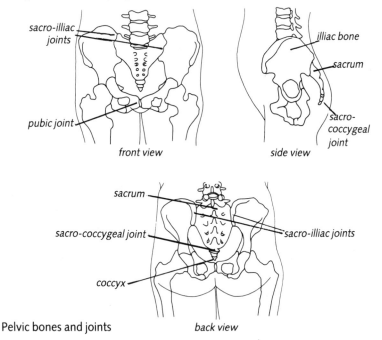

sacro-illiac joints

pubic joint

front view

illiac bone

sacrum

sacro-coccygeal joint

side view

sacrum

sacro-coccygeal joint

sacro-illiac joints

coccyx

Pelvic bones and joints   *back view*

The pubic joint in front can open by as much as half an inch during labour to make room for your baby's head.

The two sacro-illiac joints are at the back. These joints expand from side to side and also move in a pivot-like way to increase the area of the pelvic canal and adapt to the shape of the descending head of your baby, as it passes through the pelvic bones.

When you bend forward, as in squatting or kneeling, your sacrum and coccyx lift up and this opens and expands the pelvic outlet. When you bend backwards or recline, this has the effect of closing the pelvic outlet and narrowing the space by as much as 30 per cent. This is one of the reasons why reclining is the worst position to adopt for giving birth.

The sacro-illiac joints

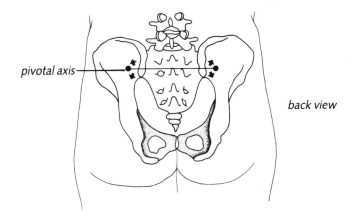

pivotal axis

back view

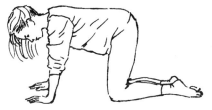

kneeling forward the
sacrum lifts up and the
pelvic outlet widens

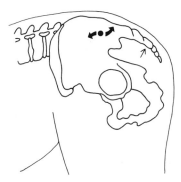

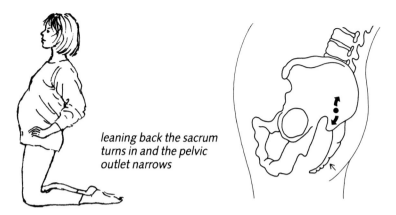

leaning back the sacrum turns in and the pelvic outlet narrows

The sacro-coccygeal joint is between your coccyx and your sacrum. This joint loosens during pregnancy so that your coccyx moves out of the way as your baby is born.

The pelvic joints are held together by ligaments which are like strips of very strong elastic.

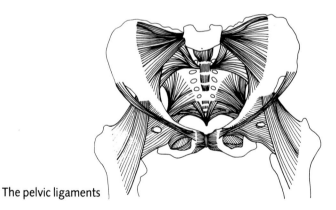

The pelvic ligaments

The sources of power of this part of your body are the muscles which are attached to the bones and bring about movement at the joints when they contract and relax. The pelvic muscles include the buttock muscles at the back which provide strength and support for your spine and upper body, and are especially important during pregnancy. At the base of your pelvis, attached to the area around the outlet, is a sling-like band of muscles which form the pelvic floor. These surround and form the base of the anus, vagina and urethra. These muscles support all the abdominal contents and your baby will pass through them as he is born.

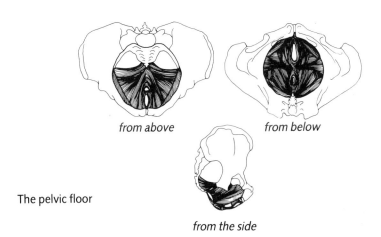

from above   *from below*

The pelvic floor

from the side

The uterus is a powerful muscle shaped like a hollow bag within which your baby is growing. It is attached by strong ligaments to the pelvic bones.

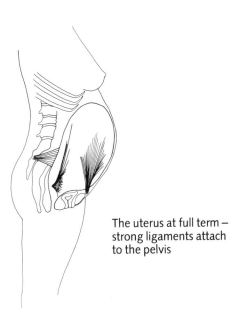

The uterus at full term – strong ligaments attach to the pelvis

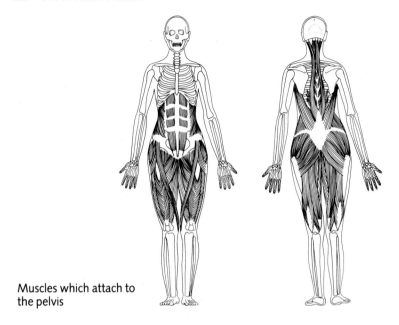

Muscles which attach to
the pelvis

Other muscles which are attached to your pelvis are the abdominal muscles, back and leg muscles. Your pelvis supports and distributes the weight of your upper body, and protects and supports your uterus and growing baby.

Correct flexion of the pelvis during pregnancy is crucial for good posture, for the safe carriage of your child and will help to ensure a good birth. The exercises for pregnancy concentrate on the pelvis and include all the major joints of the body.

Your Spine During Pregnancy

Your spine is made up of a column of bony vertebrae which extends from the coccyx or tailbone at the base, and includes the fused vertebrae which make up the sacrum (back wall of the pelvis), then the vertebral column which begins with the first lumbar vertebra in the lower back, and continues all the way up your back to the smaller vertebrae, which make up the neck and support your head. In the joints between the vertebrae there are spongey discs which act as shock absorbers and assist healthy movement of the spine.

The spine has natural curves and is capable of a range of versatile movements. A healthy spine can bend backwards or forwards, it can twist or go from side to side, or it can combine several of these movements at the same time. Your spine is the central shaft of your skeleton and supports your internal organs, your ribs, and lungs, as well as your head. It contains your spinal cord and is the supportive structure of your autonomic nervous system. It controls movement and keeps your body weight balanced. Your spine is dynamic at all times – even when you are asleep.

During pregnancy your spine has the additional task of supporting the weight of your growing uterus and its contents. As your baby grows, the natural curves of your spine will adjust to the additional weight in the front of your body. After your baby is born your spine will regain its normal curves and will have to cope with the many hours of carrying your baby during infancy.

A healthy spine should adapt easily to the demands of pregnancy and mothering.

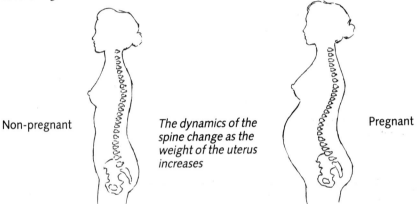

Non-pregnant

The dynamics of the spine change as the weight of the uterus increases

Pregnant

However, often we are unaware of underlying imbalances or stiffness in the spine, and the additional stress of pregnancy may result in poor posture and back pain. Practising the exercises in the next chapter regularly will help to relieve or minimise back pain and will strengthen your spine and help to maintain its flexibility.

Heart and Lungs

During pregnancy your fluid and blood volume increases considerably to ensure that sufficient blood is pumped to and from the uterus and placenta, as well as the rest of your body. Your heart works harder and your breathing changes as well. In order to nourish and carry your baby well, your whole body works harder than usual.

As pregnancy advances the extra weight you are carrying may make it more difficult to exercise and exert yourself in the usual ways. Yet, with birth and motherhood ahead, it is important to maintain or improve your fitness in the right way. Appropriate non-strenuous exercise will help to keep your cardiovascular system at its best, and ensure that you are breathing well and that the blood going through to your baby is well oxygenated.

3 | Yoga-based Exercises for Pregnancy

During the nine months of pregnancy your body will need to accommodate enormous physiological changes. New demands will be placed on your system as you breathe, digest and excrete – not only for yourself but also for your growing baby.

In early pregnancy, you will be adapting to the hormonal, physical and psychological upheavals that are common at this time and may need to cope with unusual tiredness or nausea. Later on, in mid-pregnancy, you will probably feel more settled and enjoy a sense of vitality, health and well-being. At this time you will want to exercise and use your body in a way that makes the most of its tranformative potential and is appropriate for pregnancy. In the last few months, as your body adjusts to the increasing weight you are carrying, you will benefit from exercises that protect and strengthen your spine and exercise your whole body without strain. You will also need to prepare for the challenge of labour, birth and motherhood.

Most of the exercises in this chapter are derived from hatha yoga and are particularly suitable for pregnancy. A few are adapted from physiotherapy to strengthen the body appropriately and prevent stress.

Yoga is an ancient system of exercise which originated in India and is now widely practised all over the world. It is a way to both relax your body and quieten your mind and to find your inner centre. Most importantly, yoga, correctly practised, educates your body to exist in harmony with the force of gravity. Without using force or strain of any kind, you can learn, with the help of your breathing, to let go of unnecessary tension and stiffness in your joints and muscles. Gradually, as your posture improves, you will feel more grounded and connected with the earth and your body and mind will find equilibrium, unity and balance. Like a tree that has firm roots extending into the earth, a stable trunk and branches that are free to blow in the wind, your body will become more rooted at its base where it meets the earth, allowing lightness and freedom in the upper body and an increasing sense of inner calm and security. This will help you, not only in pregnancy, but will extend very naturally into labour and birth itself, without the need to learn any complicated techniques or to remember anything mentally.

In the preceding chapters, we have seen how the normal physiology of the birth process can best take place when you position your body in harmony with gravity. Each time you practise the exercises recommended in this chapter, you will be increasing your instinctive body sense and this will continue to be your guide during labour and give you confidence and faith in your own potential and power.

It will be easier to be in touch with your primitive instincts and to let go of the fear and tensions that can inhibit the involuntary birth process. You will know how to centre yourself and accept both the pain and the change of consciousness which occur as your body opens up to give birth.

Yoga can help you to flow with the challenges and transformation of pregnancy and birth from the very beginning. It will bring you greater self-awareness and will also increase your awareness of the presence of your child inside your body. You will discover, in the silence of inner peace, that it is possible to communicate with your unborn baby and to be aware of the powerful psychic and emotional link which exists between you from the very beginning. Yoga is a way to spend time with your innermost self, and to experience the oneness and creative energy of the universe. It will help you to be aware of the miracle of creation taking place within and through your body, so that you can nourish and welcome your baby in a spirit of celebration and love.

How does yoga work?

Practically speaking, yoga provides a system of exercises to help you recover the natural range of movements your body is designed to make, in harmony with the force of gravity, and to maintain structural fitness (see Recommended Reading).

In our modern technological society, most of us are victims of a hidden epidemic of muscular stiffness which inhibits our potential for movement at the joints and throws our posture off balance to a greater or lesser degree, so that our bodies are fighting gravity rather than existing in harmony with it. This results in any combination of structural imbalances such as tight shoulders, protruding head and neck, exaggerated spinal curves, rigid pelvis, stiff legs, etc., and the inevitable headaches, backaches, and other aches and pains which accompany them.

This state of affairs is brought about by the stresses and strains of modern life, sedentary life styles, loss of contact with nature, poor postural habits and physical education, and the suppression of emotions which are commonplace in our society. Most of us, without ever being aware of it, end up carrying a load of unnecessary tension around with us, actually bound up in our muscles and joints. Without our knowing it, this limits our physical and mental potential and separates us from our instinctive selves. Yoga gets to the root of tension in the body and gives us an opportunity to breathe, let go and release it. It is a fundamental approach to relaxation which has tremendous transformative potential and power at any time, but it is particularly appropriate in pregnancy.

While some yoga positions involve a complex combination of movements which affect different parts of the body simultaneously, a simple forward bend will help us to understand how the underlying mechanical principle of yoga-based exercise works.

A forward bend is a positional exercise to encourage passive relaxation of the hamstring muscles at the back of the legs, while the body is positioned to allow maximal movement of the hip joints in relation to gravity.

TRY THIS:

Stand upright with your feet about 12 inches apart and parallel. Allow your weight to settle down into your heels as you exhale, until you feel your feet are well grounded. Now, without bending your knees, bend forward slowly from your hips keeping your spine straight.

Hold for a few seconds, breathing deeply, and then come up slowly.

You no doubt felt a stretching sensation in the muscles at the back of your legs as the movement caused them to lengthen and relax. You are probably wondering why this was painful, if the muscles were relaxing. The reason is that it is so long since you have made the full movement that the hamstring muscles at the back of your legs have shortened and lost their elasticity, restricting your ability to move forward.

Nature has designed your body to be able to fold over like a jack-knife, with your stomach and chest flat against your thighs and the palms of your hands on the ground in front of you. Of course, during the later months of pregnancy, this can only be done with legs apart to make room for your belly! (See page 56.) In this position your feet are firmly grounded and gravity draws your trunk forward with a hingelike movement from the hips. Your spine should be completely passive and relaxed while the front of your body contracts and the hamstring muscles lengthen and extend.

Breathing deeply while in the position allows you to release the tightness you feel until eventually you can make the movement with greater ease.

You will probably find, as you experiment with other movements, that this state of chronic tension exists throughout your body to some degree, affecting some areas more than others. The most effective way to become more relaxed and supple is by beginning to make the neglected movements we were designed by nature to make. It is simply a matter of spending some time each day practising them. Gradually stiff muscles will lengthen and regain their elasticity, and joints will become more mobile as tension is released.

The programme of yoga-based exercises that follows will cultivate relaxation and flexibility in a safe, passive and non-strenuous way, which harnesses the help of the forces of gravity and your natural potential for movement. Pregnancy is a unique and marvellous time to let go of habitual tensions and to allow your body to become more open and relaxed.

'I'd never exercised before and found some of the positions quite hard to start with but gradually, with practice, I loosened up. I concentrated mainly on about six or seven exercises which I tried to do every day.'

The benefits of yoga-based exercise

- As your muscles become more elastic and your joints more supple, the balance of the muscle-pulls that support and move your body improves. Muscles work in teams – while one team is relaxing and lengthening, the other is contracting and shortening. By balancing the opposing teams of muscle-pull, your joints articulate better and your posture automatically improves. This ensures that you are carrying your baby correctly and will help to prevent backache.

  'I found that the most comfortable ways to rest, watch TV or read were either to sit in the tailor position on the floor or on all fours leaning on cushions. The latter position was invaluable whenever I got backache.'
- Breathing well depends on good posture. When your pelvis and spine are in good balance and your shoulders are relaxed, your chest cavity can expand easily so that breathing is not restricted. This ensures good oxygenation of the blood to nourish both you and your baby throughout pregnancy.
- As you become familiar with the exercises you will find movements which alleviate the minor discomforts of pregnancy, such as heartburn, pain in the hip joints or in the ribs, cramps in the legs or headaches.
- Your circulation depends upon your muscles. Blood vessels run through your muscles acting as pumps and return blood from your lower body back up to your heart. If a muscle is stiff then the blood vessels running through it are constricted and your blood circulation (and indeed, indirectly, the circulation to your baby in the womb) will be restricted. The exercises help to ensure that your baby is getting everything he needs to grow healthy and strong. Problems associated with poor circulation – varicose veins, haemorrhoids (piles), or fluid retention – will be prevented or improved. Yoga tends to lower the blood pressure and can often help to prevent problems associated with rising blood pressure. (See Chapter 11.)
- Yoga helps to combat fatigue. If muscles are stiff and movement is restricted, the flow of energy is 'blocked'. After a session of exercise you will feel invigorated and refreshed, and more alive. Over time this will increase and your pregnancy can be a time when you feel healthier and more energetic than ever.
- The most comfortable positions in pregnancy will naturally extend into the labour itself. So, without needing to think about it very much, you will have cultivated ease and comfort in the natural positions for birth used by women through the ages. You will be able to move freely and instinctively like a

primitive woman – your body will know what to do. Yoga will help you to be more deeply in touch with your own centre. It will be easier to behave involuntarily, and to surrender to the powerful forces within your body during labour.

'When the contractions became very strong I knelt upon the delivery bed and leant over a very large firm cushion – this seemed to be a natural position for me to adopt as I had used it so much in late pregnancy.'

'Yoga prepared me to relax as much as possible during and between contractions, to stay squatting, and to give birth in a position which allowed me to let go.'

- As stiffness lessens, you will be helping your body to become free of pain. You will learn how to become familiar with the discomforts and even the pain of going beyond your usual limits. As your labour and birth demand going beyond your normal limits, positioning your body to do this physically during pregnancy prepares you gradually for this, so that when the time of labour arrives you are familiar with this kind of effort. Yoga teaches you to surrender to the forces within your body. This is the best possible practice for labour and will help you to cope with the intensity of the sensations of your contracting uterus.

'By exercising, I learned how to be at one physically and emotionally with the changes which would inevitably lead to the birth of my child. The teaching enabled me to "go with" my body, even when the pain was a burden. I was physically and also theoretically prepared for everything that was to happen to me and I approached the final events with excitement and real confidence.'

- Whatever happens during labour and delivery, even if complications arise, practising yoga throughout pregnancy is the best way to prepare for a speedy recovery and return to normal.

The exercises

INTRODUCTION

Choose a time of day when you have an hour to yourself – first thing in the morning or perhaps last thing at night. It is best not to eat a large meal beforehand.

You will need a carpeted space with one free wall, two pillows and a low stool or pile of large books.

The exercises are arranged in eight sequences which include six basic exercises to be practised daily (these are starred and labelled 'Basic' I–VI). The whole programme should take about 1½ hours to complete but you may devise your own personal programme concentrating on the basics and then adding others according to preference or need.

For best results, start doing these exercises as early in your pregnancy as possible – any time after the twelfth week, unless your doctor advises you that it is all right to start sooner. However, it is never too late to benefit.

Start off in any easy way, holding each position for as long as you are comfortable, gradually lengthening the time as you become familiar with the movements. Start with a few of the movements and gradually build up until you are able to go through the full programme. The first thing you may feel when you start is your own stiffness, so expect to spend two or three weeks getting to know the exercises. Gradually, as you loosen up, the movements will become pleasurable.

You will probably find that some of the movements fit comfortably into your daily habits, that there are some you can practise while watching TV, reading or talking to friends, and some you would like to concentrate on. All the exercises are perfectly safe for pregnancy and, once they are familiar to you, you may safely spend longer periods in each position. If any exercise is uncomfortable after you have tried it out for a while, then leave it out and concentrate on the others.

At first you will find that, following the instructions carefully, you can go up to a certain point and then you begin to feel the stretch. In each position, reach this point and stay with it, breathing deeply, until the stretching sensation eases. Gradually your range of movement will increase and your body will become more flexible and relaxed.

'The exercises I had done during pregnancy were invaluable and made such a difference to the birth and after. I felt more confident and in control of my body and, as I write now, I realise what a benefit they have been in getting back to shape afterwards.'

A WORD OF WARNING:

Anyone can benefit from yoga, whether you have exercised before or not. However, if you have a chronic back problem or any complications in your pregnancy, such as a history of miscarriage or cervical stitch, then do check with your doctor first and follow the cautionary notes carefully.

Osteopathy is an ideal compliment to this sort of exercise and it is advisable to consult an osteopath who specialises in pregnancy if you have a back problem, pain in the sacro-illiac joints, tension headaches, sinusitis or any joint pain (see Useful Addresses).

Practising these exercises will help to relieve cramps in the calves, backache, varicose veins, haemorrhoids, high blood pressure, sleeplessness, tiredness, nausea and other common complaints of pregnancy, but do read the instructions carefully before you start each exercise.

Some women find that they are uncomfortable lying on their backs during pregnancy, particularly in the last month. This is because the weight of the heavy uterus presses on the large blood vessels in your abdomen which slows down your circulation and can cause dizziness. If this happens to you at any stage, then roll over onto your side, come up onto your hands and knees (all fours) and, in future, leave out any exercise which involves lying on your back. However, for most of us this is no problem and lying on the back for short periods, provided the knees are bent or the legs up, is very relaxing.

Similarly, some women find that the standing positions or forward bends should not be held for too long, while others enjoy holding them for a few minutes. At all times, let your body be your guide and stop to rest when you have had enough.

USEFUL TIPS

- It is important for your well-being and that of your baby that you attend regular antenatal check-ups with your midwife, doctor, clinic or hospital, as well as doing these exercises.
- During your pregnancy wear flat-heeled shoes and also use a low stool or a pile of books for squatting on, or sit on the floor cross-legged instead of on a chair whenever possible.
- It is a good idea to get together with another friend who is pregnant, or perhaps a small group, and practise together. Some of the exercises include partner work; they are equally beneficial for men, in case your partner wishes to join you.
- It can be very pleasant to follow your stretching session with a warm bath or shower, or perhaps a swim.

Exercise Sequence I

GETTING CENTRED

1 Basic Sitting
(Until you are familiar with this exercise it will help if someone reads the instructions aloud very slowly.)

Sit with your back supported by a wall.

Draw one foot in towards your body and then place the other comfortably in front of it or else sit cross-legged. Make sure your sacrum is right up against the wall.

Now close your eyes and release the back of your neck and shoulders by bringing your chin down a little, towards your chest. Focus your awareness on your breathing. Without altering your normal breathing rhythm, simply observe the breath for a few moments. As you breathe, become especially aware of the exhalations.

Feel the way your sitting bones contact the floor. With each exhalation, have a sense of dropping your pelvis downwards towards gravity, relaxing and releasing your knees, hips and legs towards the floor. Release your sacrum downwards so that all of your lower body is well 'grounded' and your back relaxed. Become aware of your spine, securely supported from the tailbone upwards, through the lower back, between your shoulders and up into the neck.

With each out-breath relax, release any tension in your eyes, your jaw, your neck and your shoulders, your belly and your pelvic floor. Place the palms of your hands gently on your lower belly, just above the pubic bone.

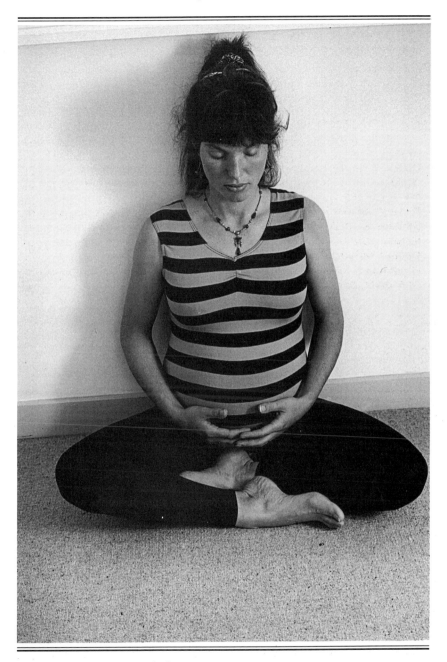

Exercise sequence I: The basic sitting position

2 *Breathing (Basic I)**

In the basic sitting position, with your awareness still focused on the breath, begin to pay special attention to the out-breath. Normally we breathe in and out through the nose but, for now, allow yourself to exhale very slowly through the mouth. When you reach the very end of the out-breath, pause for a moment or two. Then inhale through the nose to gently fill the empty space created by the exhalation.

Continue breathing like this for a few moments, keeping your body completely relaxed. Allow the breath to simply flow at its own pace. The exhalation should be approximately twice as long as the inhalation.

Continuing to breathe deeply, out through the mouth and in through the nose, bring your awareness down to the lower belly. See if you can feel the gentle movement of the belly with the breath. As you exhale, pressure in the abdomen decreases and your belly should move away from your hands towards your spine. Pause. Then as the breath comes in, pressure in the abdomen increases and your belly should expand towards your hands.

Continue breathing like this, feeling the belly withdraw away from your hands with each exhalation and expand gently towards your hands, as the breath comes in.

The rest of your body should remain relaxed and still, with very little movement in the chest and shoulders.

When you breathe deeply you are mainly using your diaphragm muscle which moves up as you exhale and down as you inhale, creating the fluctuating pressure in the belly. When we are relaxed we naturally breathe abdominally. However, when we become tense or anxious our breathing usually rises and becomes shallow, with most of the movement happening in the chest rather than the belly, and the emphasis on the inhalation rather than the exhalation (see Chapter 4, page 79).

Many of us, without knowing it, breathe habitually into the chest rather than the belly. If this is the case, keep focusing on the out-breath and try exaggerating the movement of the belly a little, actually drawing the abdominal muscles away from your hands as you exhale, then release them towards your hands when you inhale. With a little practice, this movement should become automatic and quite natural as your breathing deepens.

Breathing with sounds will help to lengthen and deepen your exhalation. After a while deep breathing becomes effortless and can be used while practising your exercises as well as during contractions in labour. When contractions intensify, releasing sound with the out-breath will help to release the pain.

Try practising deep breathing with your partner. He can help by sitting beside you and placing one hand on your lower belly with the other resting gently on your lower back. As you exhale, gentle pressure from his hand in front can remind you to 'empty' your belly. As you inhale, breathe in towards his hand.

Make some simple sounds out loud with the exhalation. Start with the sound 'ooo' (as in *you*). Feel the sound coming from the very base of the pelvis and continue until the end of the exhalation. Then pause and let the in-breath come in as usual. Repeat the sound 'ooo'.

Then try the sound 'aaw' (as in *saw*), feeling the 'aaw' sound coming from the belly and repeat twice.

Now try the sound 'ah' (as in *far*), coming from the heart or chest.

End up by humming as you exhale.

Now place your hands palms up on your knees and, with your eyes closed, keep your awareness focused on your breathing, returning to your normal breathing-in and out through the nose.

Using sounds as you breathe out will help to lengthen and deepen the exhalation and will also help you to overcome inhibition about releasing sound during labour and birth.

3 Meditation and baby awareness

Sit quietly for a few moments, your awareness on the rhythm of the breath bringing you more and more deeply in touch with your own centre. If thoughts or distractions arise, simply acknowledge them and then bring your concentration back to the breath.

Then focus your awareness on the presence of your baby, sheltered inside you. Imagine for a moment what it must be like for your baby to be inside your womb. Imagine the feeling of the warm amniotic fluid on your baby's skin. Imagine the sounds that your baby can hear – your heart beating day and night, the food moving through your digestive system, the air whooshing through your lungs and the blood pulsing through the placenta and the umbilical cord.

From early pregnancy and especially in the last few months, your baby can hear the sound of your voice and other sounds from outside like music or the voices of other family members. He or she may also be sensitive to your thoughts, dreams and feelings as well as your touch, as you stroke and massage your belly every day. Allow yourself to become aware of your ability to communicate with your baby, and spend a few more quiet moments together before slowly opening your eyes.

You are now ready to start the exercise programme.

Exercise Sequence II

PELVIC RELEASE

1 Tailor Pose (Basic II)*

Sit against a wall with your lower back touching.

Bend your knees and place the soles of your feet together with the outside edges touching and the soles opening out like the pages of a book.

Hold your feet for a moment with your hands and stretch up and straighten your spine. Now let go of your feet and allow your knees to relax and open towards the floor.

Breathe comfortably and deeply. With each exhalation feel how your sitting bones contact the floor and release your lower back and pelvis downwards towards gravity. With the inhalation feel your spine become longer and lighter, remembering to keep your shoulders, head and neck relaxed and your pelvis grounded.

Feel the hip joints relax and release, tension melting towards the floor, allowing your pelvis to feel more and more grounded as the upper body lightens. Hold for a few moments, releasing and opening into the posture with your breathing.

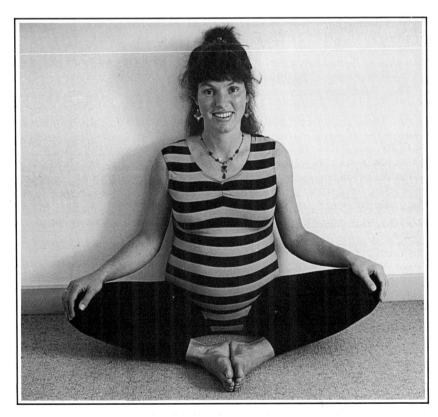

Exercise sequence II, no. 1: Tailor pose

Advanced Posture

If your legs are resting on the floor, hold your feet and, with a completely straight back, bend forward from the hips, keeping your pelvis well grounded. Go only as far forward as you can manage without bending your back. If the forward movement is easy then place your hands palms down on the floor in front of you and go down as far as your belly will comfortably allow.

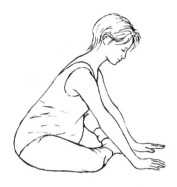

Advanced tailor pose

Benefits

This exercise releases tension in the hips, groin, knees and ankles, and helps to widen the pelvis and correct posture. It relaxes the pelvic floor and improves circulation to the whole area. It should be practised daily and can be used for short periods as a sitting position. Known as the 'woman's posture', regular practice is said to promote gynaecological health and good function of the pelvic organs.

2 Ankle Release (not illustrated)

From the tailor pose, stretch your legs out together in front of you and extend your heels. Feel the stretch along the back of your legs and then point your toes. Repeat twenty times, alternating heels and toes and bringing the back of your knees towards the floor. Separate your legs a little and rotate your ankles making circles, first inwards and then outwards. Do 20 each way.

These exercises loosen the ankles and improve movement in the joints.

3 Knee Bend

Now bend your right knee and place your right foot on the left thigh, bringing it up towards the groin as far as you can comfortably manage.

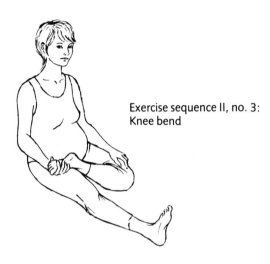

Exercise sequence II, no. 3:
Knee bend

Stretch your left leg out in front of you and extend your heel feeling the back of your leg contact the floor. Place your right hand on your right knee and breathe deeply, releasing towards the floor with each exhalation, feeling both sitting bones contact the floor. Hold for a few moments and then repeat on the other side, extending your right leg and bending the left. Hold for a few moments.

Then, release the left leg, bend the knees and place both feet together again in tailor pose. This exercise will help to reduce stiffness in the knees, hips and ankles.

4 Legs Wide Apart

Making sure your lower back is still in contact with the wall, spread your legs apart as wide as possible. At first, let your legs be heavy and floppy and breathe deeply, grounding your pelvis with the exhalation.

Keeping your thighs heavy, stretch your calf muscles and slowly extend your heels so that the back of your knees move down towards the floor.

Work with your breathing, exhaling towards gravity and grounding the pelvis and the back of the legs. Allow your spine and upper body to lengthen and lighten with the in-breath, keeping neck and shoulders relaxed.

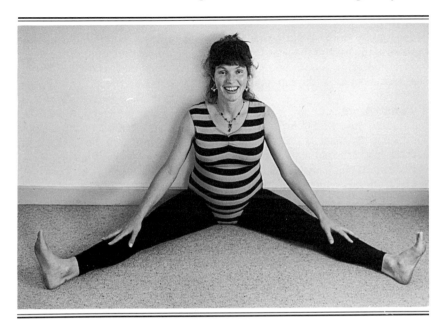

Exercise sequence II, no. 4: Legs wide apart

Advanced Posture

If you are able to, lean forward gently, moving from the hip joints and keeping your spine absolutely straight, pelvis grounded, neck and shoulders relaxed. Go as far as you can comfortably manage, without bending your back with your palms or even your elbows (or hold your ankles) on the floor.

End by bending your knees and returning to the tailor pose.

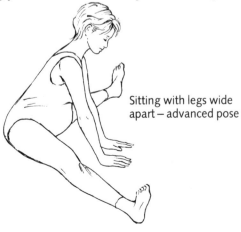

Sitting with legs wide apart – advanced pose

Benefits

This exercise widens the pelvis while releasing tension in the hamstring muscles at the back of the legs. It relaxes the pelvic floor and grounds the lower body encouraging release and relaxation in the spine, neck and shoulders. It increases mobility of the hip joints.

5 *Partner Work*

Sit in tailor pose with your partner sitting behind you, let him or her support your spine by placing the soles of both feet against your lower back or, alternatively, one foot above the other along the spine. This will prevent your pelvis from tilting backwards and your spine from 'collapsing'!

Hold for a few moments and then change to sitting with legs wide apart, alternating as you please.

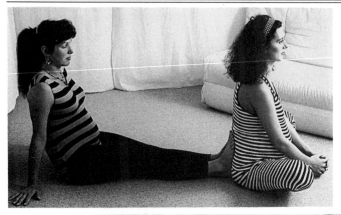

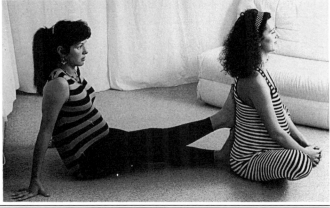

Exercise sequence II, no. 5: Tailor pose with partner

Exercise Sequence III

KNEELING POSITIONS

1 *Kneeling with Knees Wide Apart (Basic III)* *

a Kneel on the floor with your pelvis resting on your heels, your knees as wide as possible and your toes pointing inwards towards each other.

With your awareness on the breath, exhale and release your lower back downwards towards your feet so that your pelvis drops down on to your heels.

b Keeping your back, neck and shoulders relaxed, your pelvis down and your spine straight, move forward from your hip joints, placing your palms on the floor in front of you.

Keep focusing on releasing your lower back downwards and sinking your weight into your hip joints.

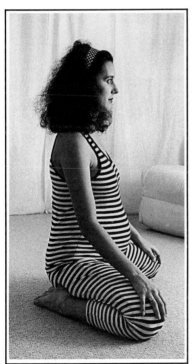 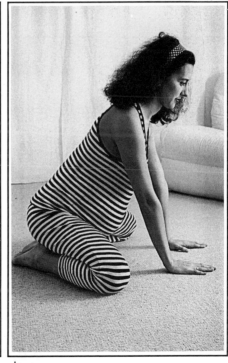

a   b

Exercise sequence III, no. 1: Kneeling with knees wide apart

(continued over the page)

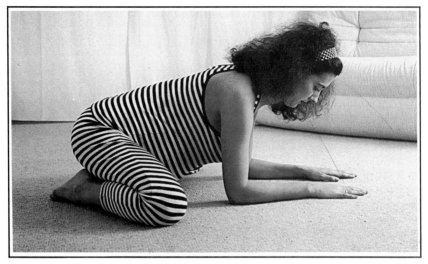

c

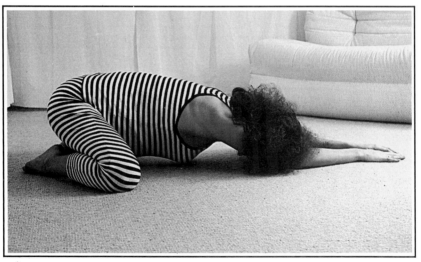

d

c With your pelvis on your heels, drop down on to your elbows keeping your spine absolutely straight. If you find this difficult, then only go as far as (b).

  Breathe deeply and rest in this position for a few moments.

  You will feel the stretch in the groin. Take your breath right into the stretch and release tightness and tension with each exhalation.

d If (c) was easy, then stretch out keeping your pelvis well grounded on your heels, your forehead on the floor and your arms stretched out in front of you. Hold for a few moments, breathing deeply and then come up slowly.

2 Partner Work

Your partner can help by placing one hand on your sacrum and gently leaning his body weight downwards to anchor your pelvis.

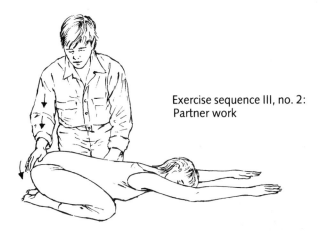

Exercise sequence III, no. 2:
Partner work

Benefits

This exercise opens and relaxes the pelvis and benefits all the pelvic organs as well as the pelvic floor. It releases tension in the inner thighs and the groin and improves circulation to the pelvic area and the uterus. It also relaxes the lower back and is especially comfortable in late pregnancy, taking the extra weight off the spine. It improves flexibility of the knees and ankles and it can be used as a movement for labour.

3 Spinal Twist (photograph overleaf)

Bring both knees and ankles together and sit with your pelvis on your heels. Release your lower back down towards your heels with each exhalation.

Starting from the hips, allow your spine to rotate gently to the right as you breathe out. Take your left hand across your body and hold gently on to your right thigh as you turn.

Without leaning back, remain upright and continue to rotate the spine, looking round over your right shoulder to include the vertebrae of the neck. Relax your eyes.

Hold for a moment or two, breathing deeply and dropping your tailbone, and then come back to the 'centre' for a moment and repeat on the other side.

Come back to the centre.

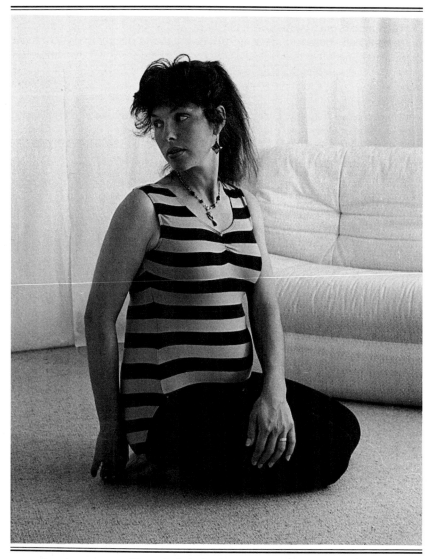

Exercise sequence III, no. 3: Spinal twist

Benefits

Twisting stimulates lubrication of the spinal joints and promotes flexibility and strength of the spinal column. It improves circulation and nourishes the spinal cord. It also releases tension in the oblique muscles of the trunk and ensures good tone of the strong ligaments that support the uterus.

4 Pelvic Lift

Start sitting on your heels with knees and ankles together. Drop your chin forward towards your chest and lean back on to your hands. Keeping your head forward and knees together, inhale and tuck in your sacrum, lifting your pelvis forward so that you feel the stretch along the front of the thighs. Hold for a few seconds then relax with the exhalation, dropping your pelvis back on to your heels.

Repeat four or five times, working with your breath.

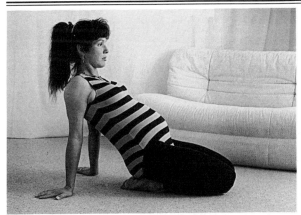

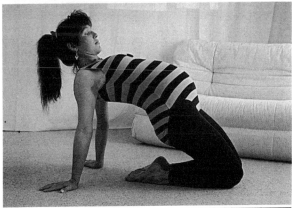

Exercise sequence III, no. 4: Pelvic lift

Benefits

This exercise strengthens your lower back and stretches the front of your thighs. It will reduce or prevent backache or pain in the sacro-illiac joints.

5 *All Fours Tuck-ins*

Come forward on to your hands and knees placing your palms and your knees about 12 inches apart.

Tighten your buttock muscles, drop your tailbone down towards your heels, tucking your pelvis under, arching you back like a cat, and then release gently. Repeat several times.

This will strengthen your lower back and alleviate backache.

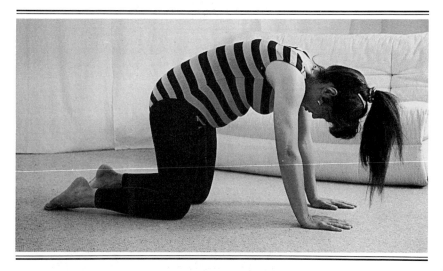

Exercise sequence III, no. 5: All fours tuck-ins

6 *Movements for Labour*

a Still on all fours, try rolling your hips around in wide circles, breathing deeply and focusing on the exhalation. Breathing out and letting go, continue for a few moments and then reverse and circle in the opposite direction. Try rocking gently backwards and forwards – exhaling towards your heels, inhaling as your weight comes onto your hands.

b Try rolling your hips in an upright kneeling position.

c Now try half-kneeling and half-squatting by bringing one knee up and rocking backwards and forwards as you breathe.

d Stand up and place your feet parallel and about 12 inches apart, your hands on your hips and knees slightly bent.

Try rolling your hips in both directions alternately, focusing on breathing out and letting go. Let your pelvis rotate like a belly dancer, keeping your upper body relatively still.

This is good practice for labour.

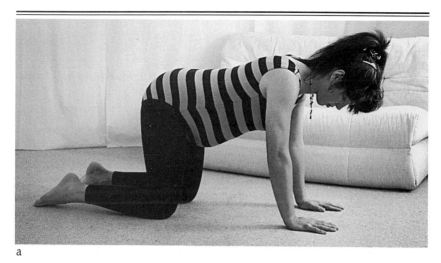

a

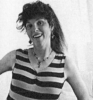

b

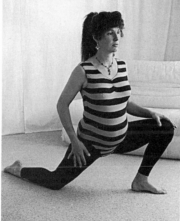

c

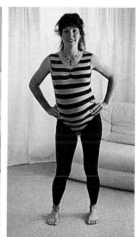

d

Exercise sequence III, no. 6: Movements for labour

Exercise Sequence IV

STANDING POSITIONS

1 Basic Standing Position
Stand with your feet about 12 inches apart. Turn your heels out so that the outside edges of your feet are parallel.

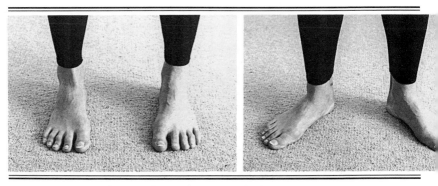

Exercise sequence IV, no. 1: Correct foot position   Incorrect foot position

Now press your big toe down on to the ground and spread your feet out wide by stretching and separating your toes. Feel the way the soles of your feet contact the ground and bring your weight to rest evenly on both legs.

Breathe evenly, in and out through the nose and, as you exhale, feel your weight dropping down into your heels so that each exhalation (like the roots of a tree going down) connects you with gravity and makes you feel more and more grounded. Lift your arches so your weight is supported by your heels, the outside edges of your feet, and your toes.

Now, with your feet firmly planted, relax and release your knees and drop your sacrum and tailbone towards your heels so your pelvis tucks under gently to support your upper body. Relax and release your shoulders and neck, and be aware of your head balanced evenly on top of the neck vertebrae.

This is the basic standing position and forms the foundation for good posture while you are pregnant. If you make sure that your feet are parallel, heels well grounded, and your tailbone drops down towards your heels when you stand or walk, you can't go wrong.

Caution: A few women feel light-headed when standing for any length of time during pregnancy. If this is the case omit this sequence or do it very gently, holding only for short intervals and resting on all fours in between exercises.

2 Warm Up

Before beginning the standing postures, stand in the basic standing position and try rolling your head around like a big, soft heavy ball to release tension in the neck.

Breathe evenly and gently, moving only your head and neck to make a complete circle, and relax your jaw.

Repeat several times, and then reverse and roll in the other direction.

Come back to the centre.

Now try rolling your shoulders only, first making circles coming forward and then reverse, rolling backwards.

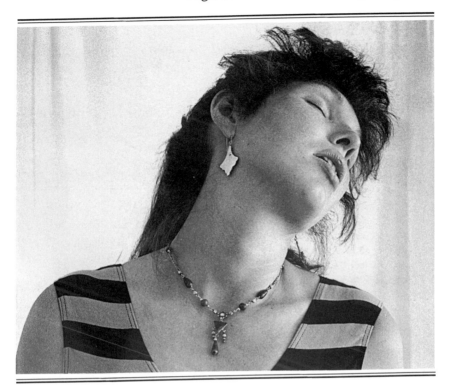

Exercise sequence IV, no. 2: Head roll

3 Pregnancy Sun Salute *(see photographs overleaf)*

a Stand in the basic standing position. Place the palms of your hands together with the wrists touching in line with your elbows, an inch or two in front of your breastbone. Become calm and centre your awareness on your breathing, dropping your weight from your lower back down into your heels. Inhale.

b Now, exhale and bring your hands down to touch the bottom of a circle.

c Inhaling, bring your arms up slowly as if you were drawing a big wide circle, then place your palms together, your fingertips touching the top of the circle. Look up at your hands.

d Exhaling, bend forward slowly and gently releasing your upper body completely and letting arms, head and neck hang forward loosely.

e Stay in this forward bend position for one more inhalation and long exhalation, dropping your weight into your heels and feeling the stretch at the back of the legs.

a–d

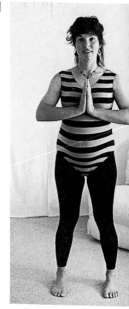

Exercise sequence IV, no. 3: Pregnancy sun salute

e–j

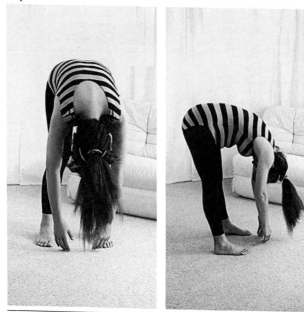

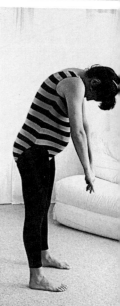

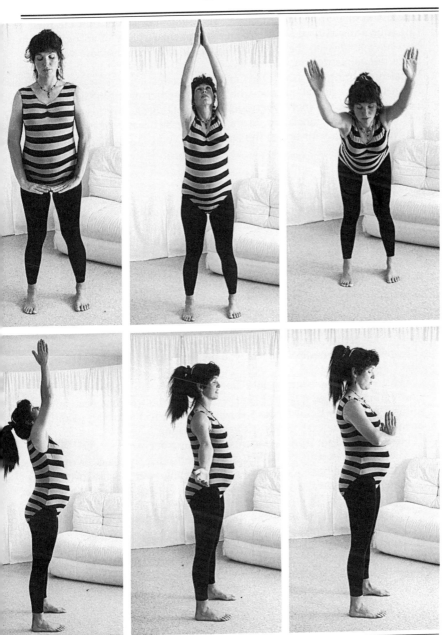

f Inhale and begin to come up slowly, uncurling your spine from the root.
g Lift your arms as if you were pulling an imaginary piece of string up from between your feet to the top of the circle, at arms length above your head.
h Place the palms together. Look up.
i Exhale and bring the arms down in a wide circle.
j Return to the original position with palms together on an inhalation.

Exhale and release your lower back and heels down towards the ground. Then, with the next inhalation, begin the cycle again and repeat about four times, working with your breath but stopping as soon as you feel you have had enough.

Benefits

This exercise is calming and centering, and invigorates the whole system, opening the chest and stimulating breathing and circulation as well as releasing tension from the hamstring muscles at the back of the legs.

This is an excellent exercise to do first thing in the morning or in between long intervals of being seated at a desk.

4 Forward Bend

(Caution: Leave this out if it makes you feel lightheaded.)

a On a firm surface, stand with your feet 3 feet apart and parallel. Turn your heels out and bring your weight on to the outside edges of your feet, lifting your arches. Grip well with your toes.

If you have a non-slip yoga mat, you may wish to take your feet wider apart (see Useful Addresses).

Exhale and drop your weight into your heels and then bend forward slowly from the hips, releasing your spine, upper body, arms, head and neck towards the floor. Bend forward slowly until you feel a stretch behind your knees and then release gently with the exhalation.

Hang forward for a few moments, breathing deeply.

Keep your feet well grounded, stretch and open the back of the knees, pointing your tailbone downwards and bringing your weight forward over your toes. Come up slowly on an inhalation as soon as you feel you have had enough.

You may prefer to repeat the movement a few times, holding for a few seconds only each time.

b If you find (a) difficult, particularly towards the end of your pregnancy when the weight of your belly increases, place your hands on a table or chair for support, forming a rectangle between your trunk and your legs.

Benefits

This relaxes and lengthens the hamstring muscles at the back of the legs and also releases tension from the pelvic floor. Helps to improve circulation and eliminate fatigue and releases the spine.

a

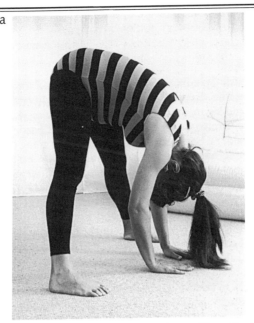

b

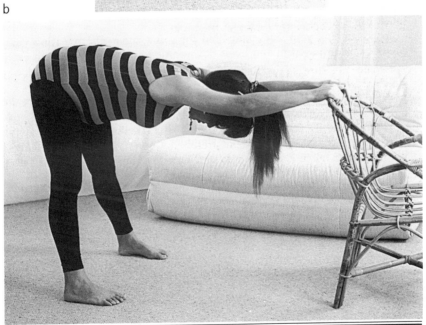

Exercise sequence IV, no. 4: Forward bend

Exercise Sequence V

SHOULDER RELEASE

1 *Shoulder Stretches*

a Stand in the basic standing position with heels and lower back releasing downwards. Breathe deeply for a few moments and, with each exhalation, allow your shoulders to drop down towards the floor. Keeping heels and pelvis going down, raise your arms gently above your head without tensing or lifting your shoulders. Sense the back of the ribcage going downwards. Clasp two fingers of one hand with the other and breathe easily, exhaling down through your ribs, sacrum and heels towards the floor. Release your arms slowly.

b Now, still in basic standing position, bring your arms gently backwards, keeping your shoulders, ribs, sacrum and heels releasing downwards with your breath, and clasp your hands. Feel your shoulder blades coming together at the back as the front of your chest opens and expands. Hold for a few breaths and then release.

c Standing in the basic standing position, roll your shoulders softly a few times forward and back to release them. Breathe and relax the shoulders and then, bending your elbow, take your left hand up the middle of your back and reach down with your right hand clasping your fingers. (If you cannot reach them, use a soft belt as illustrated [d].)

    Avoid arching your back and hold for a few moments, releasing your shoulder blades, sacrum and heels downwards towards the floor with each exhalation. Your top elbow should be pointing at the ceiling, your lower elbow to the floor. Release and repeat on the other side.

e Kneel with knees wide and your buttocks on your heels, facing a wall. Breathe deeply and, with the exhalation, release your pelvis and thighs towards the ground and then stretch your arms up gently over your head and place your palms on the wall at a shoulder's width apart, spreading your fingers. Tuck under your pelvis so your sacrum drops towards your heels and your lower back remains relaxed. Keep your palms as high as possible and your elbows straight if you can. Each time you breathe out, release your chest towards the floor without moving your hands. Hold for a few breaths and then come up slowly. You should feel this stretch in the upper arms and shoulders. Repeat once or twice.

Benefits

These exercises relax and release the shoulders and the rib cage and increase the capacity of your chest cavity. They will help release pain which commonly occurs in the ribs in late pregnancy, relieve or prevent tension headaches, and improve your breathing and posture. While pregnancy exercises tend to place emphasis on the pelvic area, it is important to work regularly on the shoulders to maintain a balanced relaxation in your body.

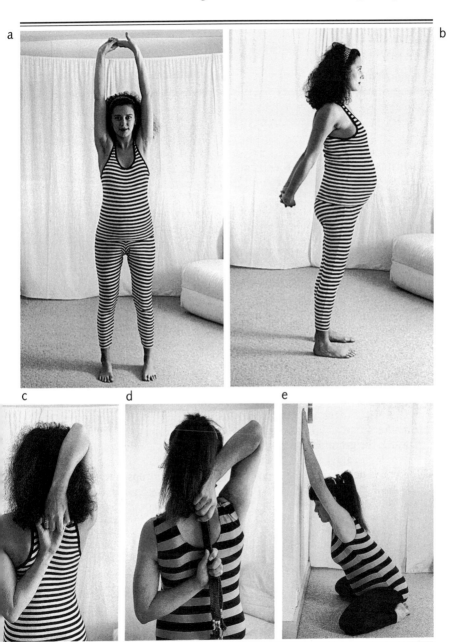

Exercise sequence V, no. 1: Shoulder release

Exercise Sequence VI

SQUATTING

1 Calf Stretch

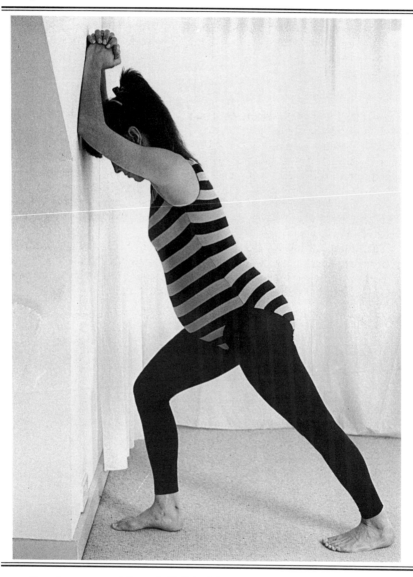

Exercise sequence VI, no. 1: Calf stretch

Stand up and, facing the wall, place your left leg in front of your right with both feet facing directly towards the wall. Bend your left knee and keep your right knee straight, then clasp your hands and lean forward, placing your elbows and forearms on the wall.

Bring your right foot back as far as you can without lifting your heel. Breathing deeply, sink your right heel into the floor with each exhalation, releasing and opening the back of the right knee. You will feel the stretch in the right calf muscle and along the achilles tendon. Breathe into it for a while and then change legs.

Repeat twice on both legs.

2 *Dog Pose*

a Kneel on all fours with your hands and knees about twelve inches apart and your fingertips touching the wall.

b Breathe for a moment or two and relax your neck and shoulders. Tuck your toes under and lift your pelvis, coming up on to your toes (see overleaf).

c Then, on an exhalation, bring your pelvis backwards and drop your heels towards the floor, placing them down on the ground if you can. Keep the back of your knees open and try to keep your shoulders and arms relaxed, with your body weight by-passing the pelvis and going down through the back of your legs and your heels into the floor.

Take a few breaths, exhaling down through your heels, and keep bringing your tailbone back towards your heels and opening the back of the knees.

Return to the resting position on all fours, relax and then repeat twice more, holding for short periods only, if you want to.

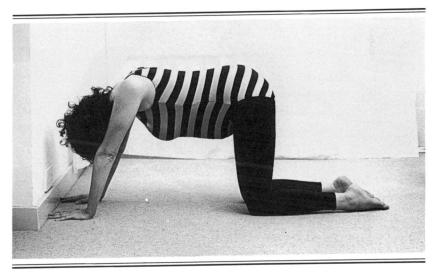

Exercise sequence VI, no. 2: Dog pose a

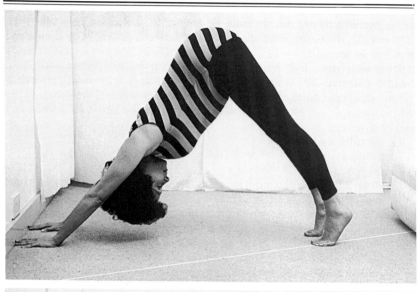

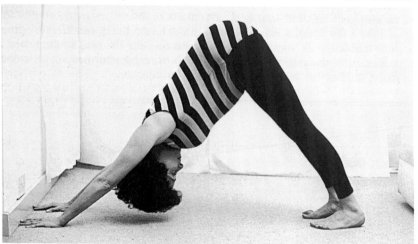

Exercise sequence VI, no. 2: Dog pose b, c

At first this exercise will probably be rather difficult and you will feel a bit top heavy. With practice, the back of the legs will become less tense and you will find it easier to have a sense of release in the shoulders when the heels become more grounded.

Benefits
These postures release tension from the hamstring and calf muscles, reducing fatigue, while improving circulation to the legs. They increase ankle flexion and thus help to improve ease in squatting. They will eradicate or improve cramps in the calves, particularly if practised just before going to bed at night.

Once you have developed greater ease in (2) you will find it a helpful way to release tension from the neck and shoulders.

3 Squatting (Basic IV: see photographs overleaf) *
a If you have haemorrhoids (piles), vulval varicosities or a cervical stitch, or if you find full squatting difficult, use a low stool or a pile of books. Do not do b, c and d.
b Start squatting with a partner if possible, or else hold on to something firm like a window ledge or the edge of your bath.

Hold each other by the wrists and stand a full arms length away from each other with elbows straight. The supporter should place one foot in front of the other with heels firmly planted, and lean back slightly to support your weight without effort or bending her back.

Stand with your feet about 18 inches apart and only slightly turned out. On an exhalation, drop your heels down into the ground, bend your knees and bring your pelvis down between your knees, holding on to your partner for support. Lift your arches bringing your weight on to the outside edges of your feet and spread your knees as wide as possible. With each exhalation relax and release your shoulders and spine and drop your tailbone towards your heels. Hold for a few breaths and then come up slowly.

Repeat once more.
c Your partner can help by standing behind you and bending forward (with back straight), placing both palms on your knees and supporting your lower back with her legs, while leaning her body weight down to help bring your weight down into your heels and spread your knees apart. Hold for a few breaths and release.

This should feel easier than squatting on your own when correctly done.
d To squat on your own, place your feet 18 inches apart and turned out slightly. With heels flat, bend your knees and place your hands on the floor, then drop your pelvis between your legs towards the ground and clasp your hands. Separate your knees with your elbows and lift the ankles. Keep your shoulders and spine relaxed and your tailbone dropping towards your heels.

Hold for a few minutes and then come up. Alternatively you may find it helpful to squat close to a wall with just your sacrum touching for support.

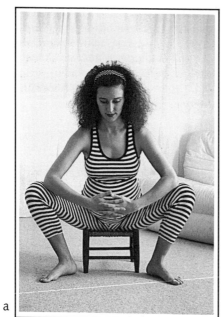

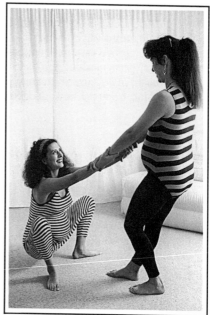

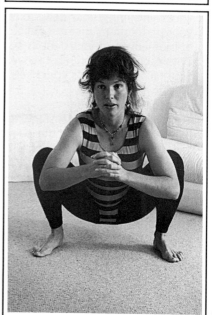

a

b

c

d

Exercise sequence VI, no. 3: Squatting

Benefits

Squatting opens your pelvis to its widest and helps to position your baby correctly and make the most of the increased flexibility and softening of the pelvic ligaments in pregnancy. It improves circulation to the whole pelvic area, prevents or eases constipation and relaxes the pelvic floor. Practising squatting regularly will help you to develop ease in the position for use during labour and birth, when you will be supported or use a stool.

4 Pelvic Floor Exercise (Basic V)*

Use the easy squatting position on your toes (below) unless you have haemorrhoids, vulval varicosities or a cervical stitch, in which case the slow-down or knee-chest position will be more helpful (see page 110).

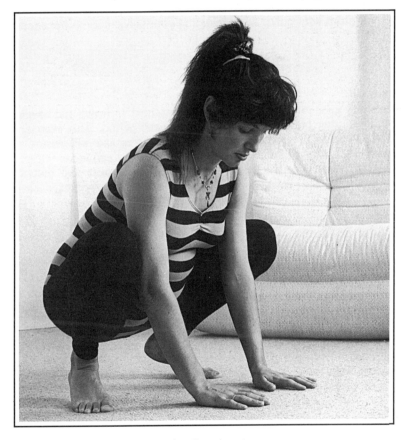

Exercise sequence VI, no. 4: Pelvic floor exercise

Close your eyes and focus your awareness on your pelvic floor – the sling of muscles that surround your vagina and anus and form the base of the pelvis. Your baby will pass through them when you give birth.

With an inhalation, draw your pelvic floor muscles upwards towards your uterus, contract, hold for a moment and then exhale and release.

Repeat several times.

Now inhale and draw the pelvic floor up. Hold the muscles tight while you exhale, then inhale again, still holding, and finally release the breath and the pelvic floor together in four little stages with a long release at the end.

Repeat twice more. This will become easier with practice.

Now try tightening and letting go quickly about ten times while breathing normally. (If you have any of the problems listed above, try doing fifty of these every morning and evening to improve muscle tone and reduce varicosities.)

It is helpful for birth to visualise your baby's head coming down and emerging from your pelvis while releasing your pelvic floor in the squatting position.

Benefits

Maintaining good tone of the pelvic floor is essential for health and happiness, especially during pregnancy and in the postnatal period. This exercise will improve circulation, prevent prolapse or varicosities and will ensure good recovery of the vaginal and perineal tissues after birth. Learning to release and relax your pelvic floor will be helpful when you give birth and reduce the likelihood of tearing. Pelvic floor exercises should be practised regularly.

Exercise Sequence VII

RECLINING POSITIONS

1 Abdominal Toner

a Lie on your back with your knees bent and the soles of your feet touching the wall. Place your feet parallel and about 12 inches apart. Clasp your hands behind your head and place your elbows on the floor. Breathe deeply into your belly and relax and release your shoulders, spine and lower back on to the floor. With each exhalation, drop the back of the waist down towards gravity. Feel the abdomen 'empty' with the out-breath and expand as the breath comes in. This is the resting position.

b Now, with an exhalation, lift your head, shoulders and arms off the floor towards your feet. Hold for a second, inhale and then exhale and release. Take a breath in and out in the resting position. Repeat six times. Then relax.

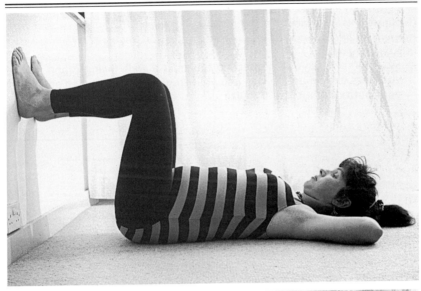

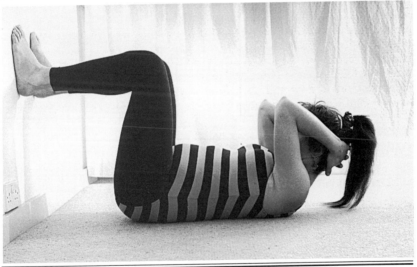

Exercise sequence VII, no. 1: Abdominal toner

Benefits
This exercise gently and safely strengthens the abdominal muscles which support your growing uterus, while your lower back is completely protected, and will prevent poor muscle tone after birth.

2 Legs Apart on the Wall (Basic VI)*

(Caution: Omit this exercise if you feel dizzy or uncomfortable lying on your back, especially in the last four weeks of your pregnancy, and concentrate on the sitting version in exercise sequence II.)

a Sit down sideways with your hip touching a wall. Swing round so that your legs extend up the wall and your trunk is at a 90 degree angle with your buttocks touching the wall.

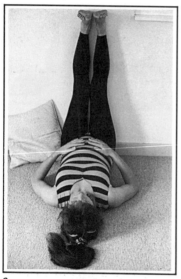

a

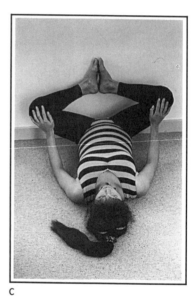

c

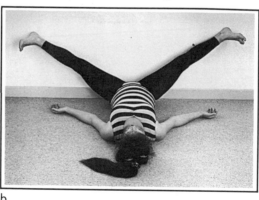

b

Exercise sequence VII, no. 2: Legs apart on the wall

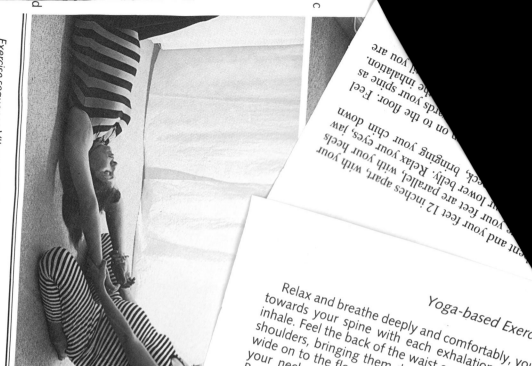

... ent and your feet 12 inches apart, with your ... s your feet are parallel, with your heels ... your lower belly. Relax your eyes, jaw ... eck, bringing your chin down ... n on to the floor. Feel ... rds your spine as ... e inhalation. ... l you are

Relax and breathe deeply and comfortably, your belly 'emptying' down towards your spine with each exhalation and expanding softly as you inhale. Feel the back of the waist contact the floor, relax and release your shoulders, bringing them down towards your pelvis and spreading them wide on to the floor. Tuck your chin in to lengthen and relax the back of your neck, and relax and release any tension in your jaw and eyes.

b Breathe calmly.

With your awareness on the back of your legs, stretch your calves and extend your heels and then allow your legs to open as wide as possible, as you exhale. You will feel the stretch in the inner thighs between your knees and your pelvis. Keep breathing deeply, dropping the back of your waist, with your knees straight. Hold for a few seconds to begin with, gradually extending the time to five minutes as tension eases.

c Bend your knees and bring the soles of your feet together close to your body. Use your hands to bring your knees closer to the wall. You can alternate (b) and (c), repeating several times.

Benefits

One of the most beneficial exercises, this releases tension from the adductors or large muscles of the inner thighs. These have an important influence on the genital area. Relaxing the inner thighs will release blocked sexual energy, improving orgasmic release in love-making, as well as giving birth. It will make you feel more open, relax the pelvic floor, and help to reduce inhibition and fear.

This should be practised daily throughout pregnancy. At first, this exercise may seem rather difficult but, after a week or two of regular practice, you will find it deeply relaxing and invigorating. Practised last thing at night after a warm bath, it will help to prevent insomnia and discomfort.

3 *Partner Work (see photographs overleaf)*

a Sitting comfortably behind her head, place your palms on her shoulders and lean your body weight forward so that you press her shoulders down, along the horizontal, towards the wall, to relax them. Hold for a few seconds and then release.

b Lift her head up, supporting the base of the skull. Encourage her to trust you and relax and let go. Then massage firmly but gently up from the base of the neck towards you, with even strokes. Alternate your hands and continue until you feel the back of her neck relax and lengthen. Then place her head gently down, pulling towards you at the same time, so the back of the neck stays as long as possible.

c Place your palms on her forehead gently and rest your finger... relax and release her eyes.
the eyelids. Relax and breathe deeply for a few mo...

d Hold her
firm but
for the l
Hold

Exercise Sequ

SPINAL RELEASE AND R

1 Basic Reclining Position

Lie on your back with your knees
heels close to your buttocks. Make su
turned out slightly. Place your hands on you
and shoulders and release the back of your
towards your chest.

Breathe deeply, dropping the back of your waist dow
the soft downwards movement of the breath in the belly tow
you exhale, then the gentle expansion towards your hands with
Continue breathing for a few moments, letting go of all tension un
deeply relaxed.

If you are not comfortable lying on your back, then omit this sequence.

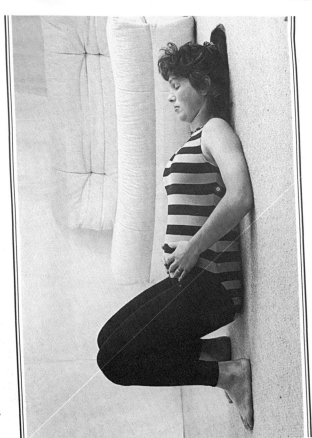

Exercise sequence VIII, no. 1: Basic reclining position

2 Pelvic Lift

Lie in the basic reclining position and place your arms by your sides with the
palms going down. Drop your heels down into the floor and then, with an
exhalation, keep your feet firm and parallel and lift your pelvis up towards the
ceiling, lengthening your sacrum and lifting your spine until your weight is

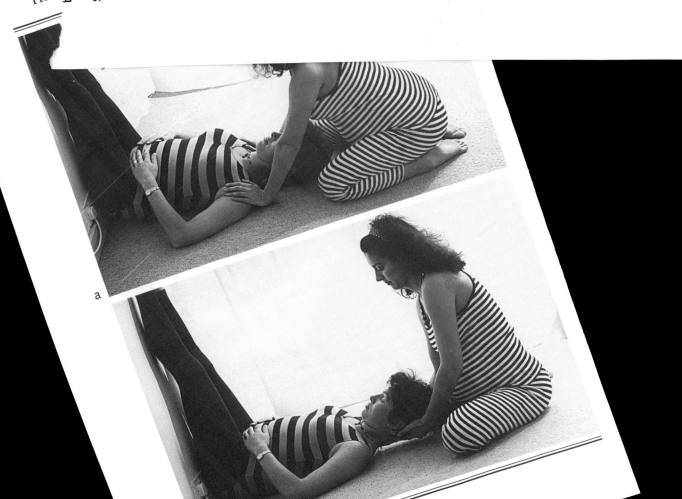

a

resting on your neck and shoulders and your feet. Keep neck and shoulders completely relaxed.

Exhale and slowly uncurl your spine releasing one vertebra at a time from the neck downwards until all of your spine is in contact with the floor once more. Take a relaxing breath and then repeat three more times.

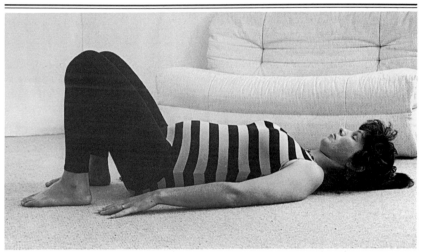

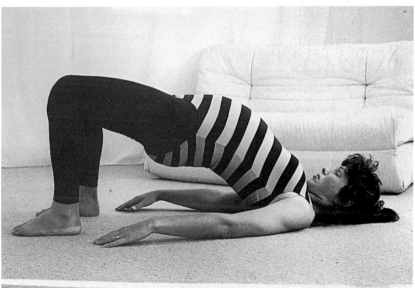

Exercise sequence VIII, no. 2: Pelvic lift

3 *Lower Back Release*

Lift your feet off the floor and draw your knees gently towards your shoulders without lifting the back of your pelvis off the floor or tensing your shoulders.

Breathe and relax for a few moments allowing your lower back to release. Now cross your feet at the ankles, place your hands by your sides and roll your hips, 'drawing' a few circles on the floor with your lower back. Come back to the centre and repeat in the opposite direction. This releases tension in the lower back and reduces fatigue.

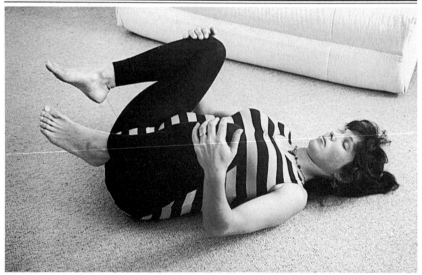

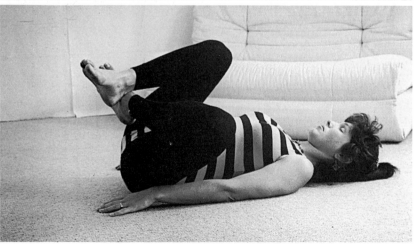

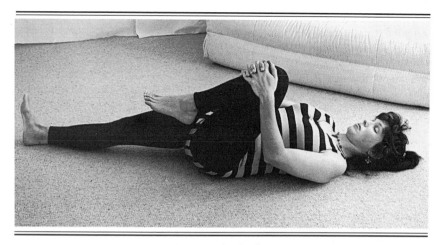

Exercise sequence VIII, no. 3: Lower back release

Extend your left leg out on to the floor and bend the right, holding the knee and drawing it gently towards your shoulder. Ensure that the straight leg is heavy and well grounded and the back of the pelvis remains evenly in contact with the floor.

The movement should be gentle, releasing with the breath, with both hips parallel.

Hold for a moment or two and then change legs.

This exercise releases and relaxes the sacro-illiac joints and will help to relieve pain.

4 Spinal Twist (see photographs overleaf)
Bring both feet together with your heels as close to your buttocks as possible. Spread your arms out to the sides so that they are in line with your shoulders. Relax and release your shoulders and spine down on to the floor and lengthen the back of your neck by tucking in your chin. Breathe deeply and, on an exhalation, turn your body to the left, bringing your knees down to the floor, while your arms and both shoulders stay in contact with the ground. Turn your head to the right so that your whole spine is rotating and twisting. Breathe and relax for a few moments and then come back to the centre.

Take a few relaxing breaths, release your spine with the exhalation towards the floor and then turn the other way – knees to the right and head to the left.

Benefits
The spinal twist nourishes, lubricates and strengthens the spinal column and releases tension in the lower back. Relieves or prevents backache.

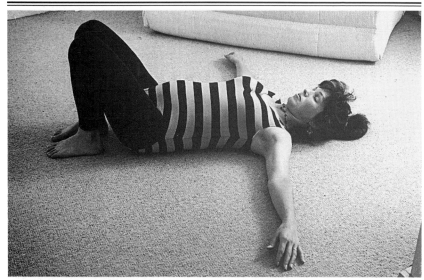

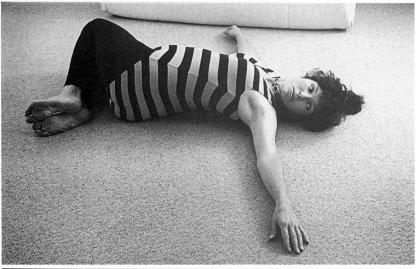

Exercise sequence VIII, no. 4: Spinal twist

Partner Work

Your partner can assist you with this exercise by sitting on your right side to begin with, and holding your right shoulder down with her left hand before you turn. Then, once you have rolled your body over to the left, she can place her right hand on your hip bone and gently assist you to turn towards the floor while keeping your shoulders in contact with the floor. It is important to do this gently without pushing, working with your breathing to let go of tension in a relaxed way.

Hold for a few moments and then repeat on the other side, with your partner on your left.

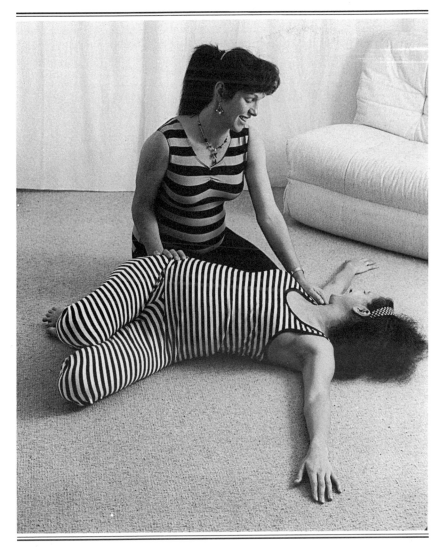

Spinal twist with partner

5 Relaxation

Place a cushion under your head and another one under your knee so that you are completely comfortable.

Close your eyes and allow all your body weight to relax comfortably on to the floor. Breathe deeply, relaxing and releasing each part of your body in turn with each exhalation.

Keep your awareness focused on your breathing and find your centre, relaxing more and more deeply.

Remain like that for 5–20 minutes. Before you come up, let your awareness go to the presence of your baby inside you and spend a few minutes in peaceful relaxation, together.

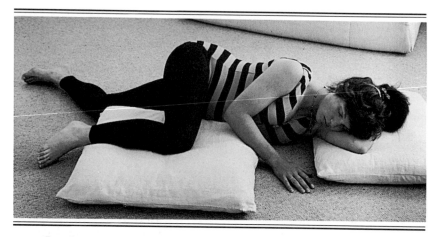

Exercise sequence VIII, no. 5: Relaxation

When you get up, take your time to open your eyes, letting the light come in slowly so that you are not in a hurry to look outwards. Keep the sense of inner peace and relaxation as you stretch out slowly and come up in your own time.

Follow your exercise session with a drink of fruit juice, mineral water or herbal tea. Avoid rushing about after exercising. Ideally, follow the session with a swim or a walk in the open air.

4 | Breathing

'The whole experience was held together for me by a combination of the upright positions and centering myself with my breathing, and "tuning in" to my body rhythms. Without this I certainly would not have had such an enjoyable time.'

This book does not include any breathing techniques. Our first aim is to ensure that you are breathing healthily (see exercise sequence I, page 38). In the same way that stiffness is a hidden epidemic in our culture, restricted breathing is another!

With our civilised way of living, our daily life rarely demands that we use our bodies to their full capacity. Many of us spend our days without physically exerting ourselves to the extent that our bodies need in order to stimulate our breathing. The result is that our breathing may become shallower and faster than it should normally be, our supply of oxygen is limited and our elimination of carbon dioxide is impaired.

If you observe the natural breathing of a baby or a young child, you will soon see that the abdomen is moving like a bellows with each breath, while the chest is relatively still and the shoulders are relaxed. This is natural, relaxed, deep breathing. By the time we reach adulthood many of us breathe too shallowly, using mainly the upper part of the chest rather than the abdomen, and approximately a third of our capacity for air. By breathing more rapidly than we should, we are taking in a new breath before we have emptied our lungs of stale air, so that we have a quantity of stale air mixed with the fresh air we breathe in, which decreases our supply of oxygen. This also decreases our vitality.

We depend upon our breathing for life and health itself – it is the basic rhythm of our bodies. Each time we inhale, we are drawing in air – the life-giving element – each time we exhale, we are ridding ourselves of waste. This constant give and take and flow of energy starts the moment we are born and continues throughout our lives, pulsating within us like an alternating current. Every other activity of the body is closely connected with our breathing.

What happens when we breathe ?

The gateway to the air passages is the nose. Tiny hairs in the nostrils prevent any dust particles from entering the lungs. The nasal passages, lined with mucous membranes, warm the air and filter out dust and germs. Glands fight off the bacteria, while our sense of smell protects us from inhaling harmful gases.

The muscles directly involved in breathing are the intercostal muscles between the ribs and the diaphragm, the strong partition of muscle separating the chest and the abdomen. The lungs themselves contain no muscles, they expand into an empty space with which they are in contact. They are enveloped by a strong membrane connected with the walls of the chest whose movements cause the lungs to change in volume as air is inhaled and exhaled.

When we breath shallowly, we are mainly using the intercostal muscles. When we breathe deeply the diaphragm muscle moves rhythmically up and down as well, allowing the thoracic cavity to expand fully.

Deep Breathing

The action of the diaphragm muscle

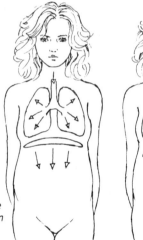

a. Inhalation
Air enters the lungs, the diaphragm moves down and pressure in the abdomen increases

b. Exhalation
Air leaves the lungs, the diaphragm moves up and pressure in the abdomen decreases

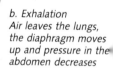

Efficient breathing depends on good posture. If your chest is tight and constricted and your shoulders hunched, the space in your thorax is less and your breathing will be impaired.

Shaped like a vault, the diaphragm muscle flattens out when it works, pressing the abdominal organs downward and the abdomen outwards as you breathe in. When you exhale it rests and arches upwards towards the chest cavity. This is what happens when you feel the movement of the breath in the belly as you breathe deeply, expanding with the in-breath and retracting with the outbreath. As the diaphragm moves up and down with each breath, this puts mild pressure on the liver, stomach and other internal organs. The rhythm of the lungs is transformed into a gentle massage which promotes the natural functioning of the internal organs. Every breath stimulates the blood circulation to these organs and increases the metabolism. This beneficial massage is lacking when we merely breathe with our upper chest.

While we can survive for weeks without solid foods and several days without water, life without air is only possible for a few minutes. Breathing is one of our most important biological functions. Every living cell absorbs oxygen and expels it in the form of carbon dioxide. If cells of the human brain are completely cut off from fresh oxygen for as little as ten seconds, the body can suffer serious harm. In pregnancy and labour you are breathing for yourself and your baby.

Breathing during labour

Normally we breathe in and out through the nose. In the deep breathing exercise (Chapter 3, exercise sequence I), part of the recommended practice is to exhale through the mouth. This is because, during strong contractions in labour, most women naturally tend to breathe out through their mouths. Make a point of breathing in and out through your nose during the day and at night, and breathe out through your mouth only when you practise the deep breathing exercise, or if you feel like it in labour or while exercising.

Regular practice of this exercise will deepen your breathing, helping you to breathe with your whole chest capacity and to use your diaphragm muscle correctly. It will also teach you to concentrate on the basic body rhythm of your breathing. Unlike the rhythm of the heartbeat, or the contractions of the uterus, which take place completely automatically, the rhythm of the breath is the only one which is both voluntary and involuntary. We are able to alter our rate of breathing consciously and this has a direct effect on our state of consciousness.

Your breathing, as you will soon feel, is very closely linked to your mind. In hatha yoga, the practice of deep breathing is a prelude to meditation. By turning inwards and focusing your attention on the breath, you will have a simple and natural tool for experiencing deeper states of consciousness. This will help you to come into harmony with your inner self and with the deep and intense feelings you will experience in labour. Focusing on the breath stills the mind, stops the internal dialogue that normally spins around in our heads and brings you closer to yourself and your baby inside. Every labour has a rhythm of its own. Concentrating on the rhythms of your breathing will help you to be at one with this rhythm, to be instinctive, to surrender to the vital forces working inside your body.

During labour there are no techniques to remember. Breathing can be spontaneous. It is now, while you are pregnant, that the daily practice of deep breathing is important. Once you are in labour you can use your ability to focus on your breath to centre yourself. You can concentrate on the exhalations and on staying relaxed through the peak of your contractions, as you can release sounds freely with the exhalation. All this will come naturally if you have learnt to breathe deeply and abdominally during your pregnancy and made this part of your exercise and relaxation practice.

'I was very aware of exactly where the baby was and how my body was doing, and people remarked afterwards how relaxed all my body had been apart from the contracting muscles. Through each contraction I used the deep breathing, at times quite fast and noisily but always with concentration and each time aware of the peak and then the fading of the pain.'

It can be very pleasant and beneficial to you both to practise deep breathing together with a partner who will be with you in labour. At first you will feel calmer and more relaxed. Gradually this will deepen to a peaceful, blissful meditation, uniting mind and body, and bringing you to your own centre, enhancing your awareness of the presence of your child within.

5 | Massage

Combined with movement, position and breathing, massage can be of great use to you in pregnancy and labour. For many people there is nothing as comforting and soothing as the touch of another. Your hands can surprise you with the magic and healing power they contain. By touching we express our love and affection for each other and we can also effectively use massage to relieve ourselves, and others, of aches and pains and unnecessary muscle tension.

Massage is an art which needs to be cultivated and the only way to learn is through exploration and experiment. There are many different kinds of massage but in this book we will explore the simplest 'intuitive' massage, without using any specific techniques.

Start on your own body, discover what feels good, which parts of your body need massage and then work with another, preferably someone who will be with you during labour. Always bear in mind that while some women love being massaged in labour and find it a helpful way of relieving pain, others prefer not to be touched. However, almost every woman will enjoy and benefit from massage in pregnancy and after the birth.

There are basically four ways you can touch for massage:

SURFACE STROKING

This is usually done with the flat of your hand. In severe pain or spasm or in a young baby or child, this very light stroking is often the only form of massage possible.

DEEP STROKING

This is done in the same way but more firmly using greater pressure.

DEEP PRESSURE

This is done by pressing firmly with the tips of your fingers or thumbs, even knuckles or elbows, over a small area at a time, getting down deep to tense spots in the body and then using small circular movements to loosen them. Deep massage works on muscle tissue and bone rather than the skin.

KNEADING

This is done by using your whole hand and alternatively squeezing and releasing a muscle and is useful over large muscle areas such as buttocks or thighs.

A good place to start is with your own hands and feet.

TRY THIS

Using one hand, explore the skin surface of the other and the bony structure underneath. Explore the range of movement of all the joints. Try feeling each finger and pressing each joint to its limit. Then separate your fingers from side to side. Now explore deeply into the spaces between the bones of the back of your hand and your wrist bones. Last, shake your hands rapidly, allowing the movement to start from your shoulders, keeping your whole arm relaxed, your wrists completely loose.

Now try your feet in the same way. Try different degrees of pressure, using your thumbs. Press all the way up the arch of your instep as firmly as you can, making small circular movements with your thumb. If you find a painful spot, linger on it for a while and try to dissolve the painful sensations. You will probably feel little crystal-like knots of tissue under the skin which yield to the firm massage and seem to disappear. Try the same thing all round the base of your big toes, the sole of your foot and then your heels and Achilles tendon, your ankles and calves. Finally explore the top of your foot and then your toes, one by one, bending them first backwards and then forwards, extending each joint to its limit. Then pull them and twist them and finally separate them from side to side.

Once you have enjoyed massaging your own feet, try treating your partner to a foot massage. You will find that your enjoyment grows and, with experience, your own natural inventiveness will lead the way.

Experiment between you with different parts of the body, neck and shoulders, back and front.

Always make sure that you are both completely comfortable.

As your interest grows you will find many good books on massage and courses are also widely available, for those who wish to go more deeply into the subject (see Recommended Reading).

Massage for Pregnancy

SELF MASSAGE

After the bath explore your whole body, perhaps oiling your skin, particularly your belly and breasts, with a good vegetable oil such as almond or wheatgerm.

In the last month of pregnancy some midwives recommend oiling the perineum with olive oil each day after your bath in preparation for birth. It will be helpful to be familiar with your pelvic area and to explore the bones of your pelvis and massage away any tension in your groin. You may want to be aware of the location of your cervix (try this gently after bathing, in the squatting position).

While you exercise, massage the part of your body where you are feeling the stretch. This is particularly useful for the inner thighs.

MASSAGE BY ANOTHER

Massage in pregnancy can be invaluable, especially before sleep and sometimes in labour. It is perfect preparation for massaging your baby after birth.

To warm up try this:

HEAD AND NECK MASSAGE

(Caution: This massage is for pregnancy but the reclining position is not suitable for labour. During labour neck and shoulders can be massaged while you are sitting upright or kneeling.)
Lie down on your back on the floor with your knees bent and legs up on a chair or bed. Place your arms down comfortably by your sides. Your partner sits or kneels behind you making sure that he too is comfortable. (Alternatively you lie down on a bed and he sits on a chair behind you.)

Press downwards on her shoulders with your hands as she breathes out to help her relax them. Now slip your hands behind her neck and stroke firmly upwards from the base of the neck towards the head, with both hands at once (see page 69). Lift your hands and repeat a few times, as if lengthening the neck. Go back over the same area but this time make small circles with your fingertips, working your way slowly up the neck.

Then lift up her head in your hands and press it slowly and gently upwards and forwards so that her chin comes down towards the breastbone in front of her chest. Hold for a second or two, and then slowly lower her head down to the ground. Now turn the head gently to one side and stroke firmly up the side of the neck, end up with firm circular movements at the base of the skull. Linger there for a while, then turn the head to the other side and repeat.

Now explore the jaw bone, the upper jaw and mouth, cheeks, cheekbones, nose, temples and the rims of the eye sockets. Make even stroking movements from the centre outwards and then go over the same area making firmer small, circular movements and exerting more pressure.

Then stroke the brow from the centre outwards and finally place your hands on either side of the head with your fingers gently covering the eyelids. Sit quietly like this for a minute, both of you breathing deeply and then gently, gently lift your hands.

BACK MASSAGE

> '*My husband gently, ever so gently, stroked the lower part of my back and this too*
> *was an enormous help.*'

Rest comfortably in the kneeling position, leaning forward onto a pile of
cushions, with your knees apart and your feet pointing towards each other. Your
partner should kneel down behind you, keeping his or her own back straight.

Alternatively, sit facing backwards on a chair, your partner can kneel behind
you on the floor or sit on a chair.

A comfortable kneeling
position for back
massage

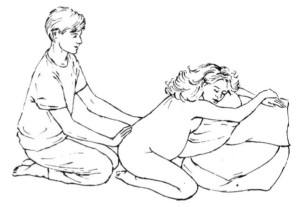

Start at the base of the skull and feel each vertebra of the spine, massaging
each one in small circles, working downwards until you reach the sacrum. Then
using the thumbs of each hand, massage the muscles on the sides of the spinal
column using as firm a pressure as your partner can enjoy, again make small
circular movements. Linger on the tense spots.

Then place your hands on the soft muscles in the shoulders and knead until
tension yields.

During labour, the lower back in the sacral area is the part that most needs
massage because the nerves which run to the pelvis stem from the lower lumbar
and sacral part of the spine. Massaging the sacrum can therefore be an effective
way of relieving pain. It is best to massage during a contraction and then to stop
in between. Use a pleasant talcum powder to avoid stickiness. Some women do
not enjoy deep pressure massage during contractions but prefer a light stroking.
Try to use slow rhythmic strokes which harmonise with her breathing. The best
way to practise this is to breathe deeply yourself while you massage. Using the
flat surface of your palm, particularly the heel, make light, slow, rhythmic
circles over the sacral area increasing pressure according to your partner's
needs.

> '*When I was in transition I became a bit panicky and here I found my husband*
> *Brian very helpful because he reminded me to keep taking deep, slow breaths. All*
> *through the contractions he gently and lightly massaged my lower back and this I*
> *found a marvellous distraction from the pain.*'

Now try using the palms of both hands and, starting at the centre, make slow even movements outwards towards or even down her thighs. Then lift your hands and repeat.

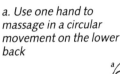
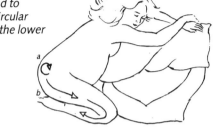

a. Use one hand to massage in a circular movement on the lower back

b. Use both hands to stroke outwards from the sacrum, down the thighs and calves

Now try to cup one hand over the lower end of the spine so that the heel of your palm covers her coccyx. Keeping your hand still, exert slight pressure so that the warmth of your hand spreads into her back. Some women find this helpful during contractions. By moving her body, the woman in labour can create the degree of pressure she needs herself.

'The heat from Ron's hand just laid on the base of my spine was so soothing and he could feel the coccyx lift.'

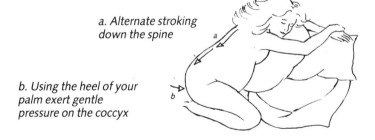

a. Alternate stroking down the spine

b. Using the heel of your palm exert gentle pressure on the coccyx

Place the palm of your left hand at the top of the spine and make a firm stroking movement down to the sacrum. Then do the same with your right hand and repeat rhythmically, alternating hands. This is very calming and can be used to quieten shivering.

THIGH, CALF AND FOOT MASSAGE

Sit comfortably on a chair, leaning forward slightly with your legs apart and feet on the floor. Your partner should kneel in front of you in a comfortable position. Using both hands at the same time, make firm stroking movements from the groin, along the inner thigh, towards the knees. Lift your hand, repeat in a rhythmical movement which harmonises with her breathing.

During pregnancy and labour, you may experience cramps in the calf muscles. Sitting on a chair place one foot in your partner's lap. Your partner should bend your foot/toes up towards your leg, take hold of the calf muscles and gently knead with his hand.

Now pass on to the foot. This can also be done in the kneeling position. During labour, foot massage can be extremely helpful, particularly in the area of the heel and the Achilles tendon, behind the ankle bones, which are said by reflexologists to influence the uterus and genital area.

Take the foot in one hand and, using the other hand, make smooth circles over both sides of the heel, and then even strokes on either side of the Achilles tendon. Explore the ankle bone and use deep pressure here to find tender spots. For some people, deep massage at the base of the ankle bone can help to lessen labour pains if you find the right spot.

BELLY MASSAGE

During labour, while you are experiencing the intense sensations of a contraction, you may find a light fingertip massage over your lower abdomen soothing. Try this yourself in the standing position.

In a half circle, make a very gentle sweeping movement over your lower belly from one side to the other. Lift your hand and repeat in harmony with your breathing.

Now try this with a partner.

Lastly, your partner should become familiar with the parts of your body which generally tense up when you are under stress, and be able instinctively to stroke away tension in labour, be it a frown on your forehead, tense, raised shoulders, clenched fists or whatever.

Many women enjoy the relaxing effect of massage in labour. However, you may find that you prefer not to be touched when the time comes, or that massage becomes too distracting. You might prefer a very light touch, or you might enjoy a deeper pressure. Make your likes and dislikes known to your partner and don't be afraid to ask for what you want as this is the only way he or she will know how best to help you.

6 | Labour and Birth

For the sake of convenience, labour and birth can be described in three stages: the dilation of the cervix or opening of the uterus is referred to as the first stage of labour; the expulsive stage – when your child is born – is known as the second stage; and the first contact between you and your baby followed by the expulsion of the placenta and membranes, is the third stage.

In the last few weeks before labour starts, you will begin to feel your uterus contracting. These pre-labour practice contractions are usually painless. You will probably feel your uterus tighten and go hard – this tightening can last for fifteen minutes or longer.

'For the last two weeks of my pregnancy I had contractions, some very strong, but after a few hours they would stop.'

At any time within the last six weeks of pregnancy your baby's head will probably 'engage' in the pelvic inlet, ready for birth. You might feel some strong contractions when this happens. Occasionally the baby's head may not engage until labour starts, particularly if this is a second or subsequent baby. Some women experience frequent mild contractions a day or so before going into labour; these can start up for a few hours and then cease and are known as pre-labour. It is important to expect the possibility of a pre-labour. If you are doubtful as to whether your contractions are the real thing, they probably are not!

The big question is – *how will you know when labour is starting?*

Established labour starts when your cervix begins to dilate. However, it can start in different ways:

1 It may start with a show, which is a discharge of blood-stained mucus, the plug which sealed your cervical opening during pregnancy. This show can come away just before labour starts or at any time during the first stage. If the plug comes away at the same time that the membranes break, the amniotic fluid may be a little blood-stained but should soon become colourless.

   'Mild contractions started about twelve hours after "the show" at five minute intervals.'

2 Sometimes the first thing to happen is the breaking of the membranes or leaking of the waters. It may come as a huge gush of amniotic fluid or a slow

leaking of the water in front of the baby, known as the fore-waters. This, too, may not happen until well on in the first stage, or, on the other hand, it can happen twenty-four hours or more before labour actually begins. Sometimes the membranes remain intact until the moment of birth. Most commonly, membranes break just before the second stage.

'I felt a "pop" and warm waters flooded out of me. I felt instantly wide awake and excited.'

'When I got up there was a trickle of water and then a show, so I knew that truly she was on the way.'

3   You may feel a persistent, dull backache which may be caused by the contractions of your uterus.

4   You may have diarrhoea as the bowels have a natural tendency to empty before labour starts.

5   You may feel very shivery and shaky. This is your body's way of letting out tension and often happens at the start of labour or at any point during labour. The best thing to do is just let it happen until it passes, breathing deeply and perhaps having your back or feet massaged.

6   The most common sign that labour has started are contractions. These will be somewhat stronger than the pre-labour contractions. They might feel similar to period pains in the lower abdomen or else you may feel them in your lower back or inner thighs.

'I became slowly aware of that familiar tightening and mild cramp in my abdomen. As I had been in a sound sleep until that point, I didn't immediately realise things had begun but as I continued to experience these pains at five-minute intervals, more or less, it was soon obvious that baby was trying to tell us something.'

The first contractions can feel quite uncomfortable or may be so mild that you can sleep through them or are unaware of them. Basically, contractions are experienced very differently by different women, or even by the same woman in different labours. They may be mild or strong when they start. They may come every half an hour or every ten minutes, or perhaps at quite irregular intervals. Your uterus will begin to contract and tighten, thinning and drawing up the cervix and then slowly opening at its base. Each contraction comes on like a wave – starting out, building up to a peak and tailing off. There will then be a rest period before the next one starts. It helps to think of waves on the shore.

Some women describe contractions as 'rushes of energy'. Anyhow, the contraction is at its strongest at the peak and can be painful at this point.

'The contractions were still very mild and ten minutes apart when I arrived at the hospital. The nursing staff were reluctant to admit me as they said I appeared to be so calm they weren't even sure I was in labour.'

'I was walking about and squatting and when I was next examined thirty minutes later they seemed to be amazed that I was progressing so quickly. The contractions were now five minutes apart and quite strong and I found that by leaning forward against the wall and also kneeling on all fours on the floor I got a lot of relief.'

As the labour progresses, the contractions become more frequent and more intense with shorter gaps between them.

By the time you are in well-established labour, the contractions will be really intense and you will need to give them all your attention.

'The contractions became a lot more demanding of me, and I mostly sat upright on the edge of my bed, leaning forward on a chair back, as I concentrated on deep belly breathing.'

'I started getting pains, rather like bad period pains. They came every ten minutes and I found that by breathing deeply through them I could easily cope with them. Between the pains I kept myself active, doing things around the house, but as the contractions got stronger I needed to rest over a pile of cushions in the gaps in between.'

The Sensations of Labour

Birth is a very special event in your sexual life as a woman. It is a time when you are transformed – you are becoming a mother, giving birth to another human being. During labour your womb will open up completely and you will also experience a change in your normal consciousness.

In the hours of labour you will want to withdraw from the normal day to day level of things and your attention will naturally turn inwards, as if the whole world contracts to what is happening within your body. In your mind, time takes on a fresh dimension. Hours can pass in what seems like minutes. It is like being in another world.

'I felt outside of time.'

'From then onwards I was centred on my body; unaware of what was going on around me.'

This great opening of the womb happens only once or a few times in your life. It is a very deep emotional experience which involves a regression to your most basic and primitive feelings, as if everything you have ever been through is part of the present time. There is, perhaps, an unconscious remembrance of once being in the womb yourself, of being born, of being a very small child, yet at the same time the dawning of yourself as a mother, and a very intimate communion between you and your body and your child within.

Your womb is the seat of your deepest feelings. In the same way that you need to sink deeply into your inner feelings when you experience full sexual orgasm, you need to respond instinctively to the urges and messages of your body when you are in labour and about to give birth.

In a way, you need to lose control, to surrender and trust in the birth process which takes place involuntarily without your conscious control. You need to let go of your mind, of everything that you know, and just let it happen. This is a time to turn inwards, to abandon oneself to the unknown, not to think ahead of what is to come, just to take it moment by moment and let the natural involuntary rhythms of your body take over.

'It's easy if you can surrender to the birth force as it passes through you. If you relax, you float; if you struggle and fight, you sink.'

You will probably experience many intense feelings of every kind, from agony to ecstasy, despair and weakness to courage and strength, from exhaustion to incredible energy and power. You are also likely to experience some nausea. Some women never do, while others experience a lot during labour. This is nothing to be afraid of and, if you allow yourself to retch and vomit, you will have immediate relief and this can help you to free yourself of tension and anxiety. Birth is a great emptying, and it is not surprising that your stomach and bowels tend to empty themselves of their contents at this time. In fact being sick can be a sign of fast dilation.

'Between those first contractions I went to the loo frequently and my baby seemed intent on a full and natural evacuation process. A few minutes later I was sick and then felt fine and ready to cope with the contractions.'

Life-giving Pain

The pain of childbirth has a bad reputation. There is no doubt about it – as any experienced mother will tell you – giving birth is painful.

It is certainly realistic to expect pain even if, in the end, you are one of the lucky few who doesn't feel any – and there are some! Most women experience pain at the peak of contractions. The pains are acute rather than throbbing and insistent, and do not generally last in between contractions. Often a very strong contraction is followed by a milder one. The pain is not the same as the pain of injury. Many women describe it as positive or life-giving pain and experience equal pleasure between contractions.

One of the main causes of unnecessary pain in childbirth is the use of the reclining position. Even if you are propped up by pillows, you are like a stranded beetle – completely helpless – and the contractions of your uterus will hurt more. Other postures such as kneeling forward, standing, squatting or sitting upright actually relieve the pain and help you tune in to what is happening inside you. You need the freedom to use your whole body to discover how to make yourself comfortable.

'I felt incredibly uncomfortable whenever I lay down and being in an upright position was basically the only way I could fully concentrate on trying to relax and keep up the deep breathing.'

'I found small movement helpful – at one point I found I was almost dancing. Leaning against anything hard was impossible for me and lying on my back was the worst thing of all.'

Often it is the wrong kind of environment and atmosphere that causes extra pain.

During pregnancy and labour your body produces hormones called endorphins which are natural painkillers that relax you and reduce pain. Another hormone secreted by your body is oxytocin which stimulates the contractions and the birth process. However, the secretion of these hormones is deeply connected with your emotions. For your body to produce them, you need to feel secure, relaxed, uninhibited and free to be yourself. The presence of other unnecessary people in the room, or someone you do not feel relaxed with, can inhibit these secretions.

'The positions had left me feeling very uninhibited and because I was at home I felt very safe and comfortable. I moaned and groaned and released the power that way too – it felt wonderful. I was an intuitive instrument for the birth – Toby was coming and my body just opened up.'

A feeling of being watched can make you tense up. These are vital considerations when choosing the attendants and place of birth. It is important for you to feel trust and confidence in the people who are helping you, to have the comfort and support of your husband or someone close to you in labour. Some women have an intense need to be alone in labour, with attendants or partner nearby in case they are needed. For some women total privacy is very important, while others need the presence of the right supporting partner close at hand.

'With constant encouragement from my husband and the midwife I felt spurred on to my goal. Ismail said afterwards that he was glad that he could help me – like bringing me back to my deep breathing whenever I lost control of it.'

We have spoken already about the change of consciousness in the first stage of labour. It is very helpful to be in a semi-dark environment at this time where there is the minimum of unnecessary sensory stimulation. Soft soothing music may help you as well as your attendants! To be able to immerse yourself in water is one of the most effective ways of relieving pain in labour. The use of a pool is ideal, otherwise have a warm bath or shower. If you feel stuck or inhibited, then try taking a bath (see Chapter 7).

'The bath was a big help and I found myself rotating my hips and massaging my tummy. I had a mental picture then of stroking and comforting the baby inside me through its ordeal. We were both, after all, in the same boat!'

There is a definite correlation between anxiety and fear and pain. When you are afraid or cold or over-excited, your body secretes adrenalin which inhibits the birth process during labour (although it may play an important part during the second stage). Your muscles tense up, your breathing becomes shallow and generally you are running away from what is happening inside you. This increases the pain. As soon as you relax and go with it, the pain lessens.

Good preparation of body and mind during pregnancy helps you to approach birth with confidence. Practising yoga during pregnancy will ensure that you are at your physical best for birth and enables you to make friends with your pain and to shed some of it before the day of the birth. Focusing your awareness on your breathing and your inner self will teach you to still your mind and to surrender to the powerful sensations inside you. The size and shape of your baby and the position in which she is lying will make a difference to the pain you feel (see page 175).

We all have differing abilities to tolerate pain. It is a very subjective experience and no two labours are alike. Some women will talk of unexpected depths of pain during labour, while others will say they couldn't really call it pain at all.

'The pain was worse than I had imagined – it was much fiercer – I felt I was being taken up by a giant hand and shaken over a raging black sea but just when I thought I was going to drown I would be pulled back by the eyes of my friend who had been through the experience already, and knew something of what I was going through.'

'I found the birth a marvellous experience – not at all painful only uncomfortable. It was marvellous being able to move about and remain upright. I felt in control most of the time.'

When birth is active, when the environment is conducive, and when the attendants are skilful, sensitive and considerate, the pain is certainly much more tolerable. In these ideal circumstances very few women need or ask for pain-relieving drugs even though these are easily available.

It is always wise though, when approaching such an unknown adventure, to keep an open mind. If you find the pain intolerable there is no need to feel any guilt about making use of pain-relieving drugs available. These do, however, enter the bloodstream of your baby and have certain side effects, which you need to consider carefully (see page 184). Some of the effects on your baby can be harmful, so do find out as much as you can about the drugs available – their pros and cons and how to make the best use of them. There are helpful homoeopathic remedies which do not have harmful effects (see Chapter 11).

Time and again I have heard mothers say, 'Even though it was painful, it was worth it!' Many women say that the moment of birth was like the greatest orgasm they have ever experienced. Women talk of great ecstasy and bliss, of the deepest feelings of joy and love. It is important to realise that the pain involved is only part of the great variety of intense feelings one experiences. If one cuts out the pain one generally cuts out, to some extent, the other feelings too.

'What a sense of completion, relief, gratefulness, and joy filled me. Similar feelings were shared by my husband and tears were running down his face.'

The greatest advantage of being able to accept and tolerate the pain, and allowing nature to take its course without disturbing the whole process, is an alert, healthy, undamaged and vigorous baby at the end of the day, and a good beginning to the relationship between you.

'This birth I found so different from that of my first baby. Then I had been encouraged to have Pethidine and I found that this made me very sleepy – not at all in control. This time, having had no drugs, I remained alert and felt very much in touch with my body although I do think that the pain was more acute.'

The First Stage of Labour

Before labour begins, your baby lies within the uterus with his or her head resting in the pelvic brim, ready to be born. The cervix or mouth of the uterus is tightly closed and sealed by a mucous plug. The membranes surrounding your baby are intact and contain the waters in which the baby floats. Before labour starts, the cervix is about 1½ inches thick and, in the week or so before the birth, hormones secreted by your body will cause it to soften and become ripe, ready to open up in labour.

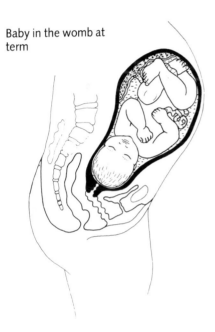

Baby in the womb at term

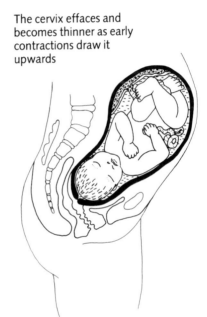

The cervix effaces and becomes thinner as early contractions draw it upwards

WHAT HAPPENS TO YOUR BABY

Before the onset of labour your baby's head engages in the pelvic brim. The widest diameter of his or her head, from the crown to the forehead, will be lying in the widest diameter of your pelvic inlet which is from side to side.

As your uterus dilates the baby's head gradually descends further into the pelvic cavity, rotating slowly as it descends. The widest diameter of the pelvic outlet is from front to back – from your pubic bone to your coccyx – which is why the baby's head rotates as it descends.

As it descends, your baby's head exerts pressure on the cervix which assists and promotes dilation. The dilating uterus pulls up around the baby's head like a glove as it goes down into the pelvic canal. By the time you are fully dilated, it will have drawn up around the baby's head as far as the ears and opened wide enough for the baby's body to pass through.

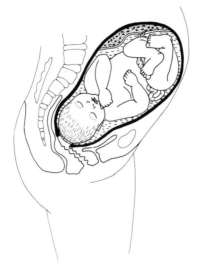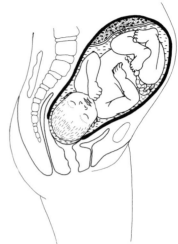

The cervix opens in early
first stage

The late first stage – the
cervix draws up around
the baby's head

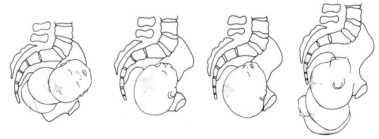

The descent of the baby's head

WHAT HAPPENS TO YOU

When labour starts the early contractions will draw up the cervix so that it thins out and becomes ready to open. Sometimes this thinning takes place in the days before labour actually begins – particularly with second and subsequent babies. You may have a pre-labour in the twenty-four hours or so preceding the birth, with mild contractions that stop and start periodically. Eventually the contractions will begin to take on a regular rhythm.

The classic labour starts with regular contractions, 20–30 minutes apart and 20–30 seconds long. After some time, as your cervix dilates, they progress to 15 minutes apart (30–35 seconds long), then 10 minutes apart (35–40 seconds long), 5 minutes apart (40–45 seconds long), 3 minutes apart (45–50 seconds long), until finally, at the end of the first stage, when the cervix is almost fully open, the contractions are 60–90 seconds long with half a minute between them.

However, very few women have such a classic labour and there is great variety in the patterns and rhythms that can occur. Some women have contractions which are 10 minutes or 5 minutes apart throughout.

The length of the first stage varies enormously, the shortest being about half an hour and the longest can be two or three days with contractions stopping at times. However, the average length of the first stage for a first birth is 8–16 hours.

Whatever the rhythm of your labour, the contractions will become more powerful, longer and closer together as your cervix progressively opens and dilates from 0–10cm (full dilation is 10cm). You or your midwife can feel the cervix dilating by vaginal examination with the hand, which is why you often hear the expression four or five 'fingers' dilated. If labour is progressing well, it is wise to do as few internal examinations as possible as they increase the risk of infection. Sometimes they are not necessary at all!

As you approach full dilation the contractions are at their most intense and you are nearing the peak of the labour.

In modern hospitals they are reluctant to allow a labour to take longer than twenty-four hours and often use obstetric means of induction (a syntocin drip) to accelerate a long labour. One of the benefits of Active Birth is that contractions tend to be more regular and efficient and labours shorter. Nevertheless it is normal for some women to dilate very slowly and, provided you have plenty of rest in between contractions and progress is slow but gradual, there should be no reason to intervene if you are coping and the baby is showing no signs of distress.

Your uterus tilts forward as it contracts, therefore it will work most efficiently and have least resistance in a position where you are upright and leaning forward.

Being in a quiet darkened room, with as few people or distractions as possible, will encourage more rapid dilation.

The uterus contracting

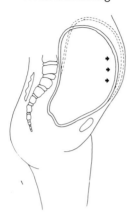

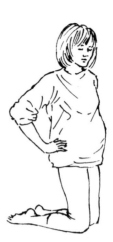

1. The uterus tilts forward as it contracts. In an upright position there is no resistance to gravity

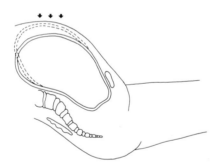

2. In the semi-reclining position the uterus works against the pull of gravity as it contracts

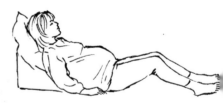

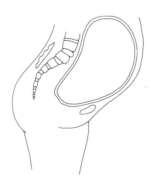

3. By standing (or kneeling) and leaning forward the uterus is helped to do its work with least resistance

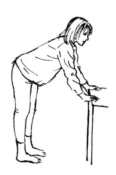

BREATHING FOR THE FIRST STAGE

Centre yourself by allowing your awareness to focus on your breathing without interfering with it, for as long as possible. When you need to, use deep breathing, concentrating on the exhalation. Try to keep your body, especially your shoulders, relaxed.

When the contractions become very intense you may need to make a lot of sound like groaning, moaning, humming, singing or even shouting. Do not try to suppress this as it is perfectly natural to do so and can be very helpful in relieving pain. Making sound causes the production of endorphin-like hormones that act as natural pain-killers and help to change the level of consciousness. It is well-known in various forms of meditation and religious worship that singing or chanting helps to still the mind and to bring one to a deeper, more concentrated state of awareness.

'As the contractions increased I found myself groaning and crying out. When the pain increased and became overpowering I still knew inside that I was in control.'

POSITIONS AND MOVEMENTS FOR THE FIRST STAGE OF LABOUR

In early labour it is a good idea to loosen up by doing some yoga (leave out the reclining positions).

Take a warm bath and just carry on with your usual activities until the contractions demand your full attention. If your labour starts at night, try to get a little sleep. It will help you to conserve your energy for the really strong labour to come. If you cannot sleep then rest in a comfortable upright position on your bed, supported by pillows.

Arrange your room so that you have a low stool or a pile of large books to squat on, something firm to kneel on, a soft mat or blanket to place under your knees and plenty of cushions with one or two large, firm floor cushions or a bean-bag. A hot water bottle may be useful. The positions shown below are the basic movements which come naturally during the first stage. Use them as a guide and change positions from time to time. Try to make yourself comfortable and, above all, let your own instincts guide you. Allow yourself a few contractions to get used to a new position. It may help to move your pelvis rhythmically during contractions, either rocking to and fro, from side to side, or in slow circles, as this will aid the dilation of your cervix, the descent of your baby and help to dissipate the pain.

'I felt the contractions so strongly that I could really only do one thing: walk, walk, walk – at quite a pace!'

Walking or standing or 'ambulation' in labour is now recognised by experts, who have done research into the subject, to shorten labour and increase the efficiency of contractions. In the early part of the first stage, try to walk about, leaning forward for contractions.

Close physical contact can be helpful during labour. The mother is supported by her partner in the standing position.

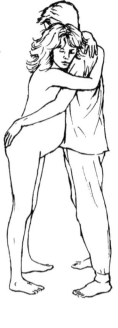

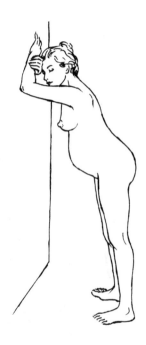

Standing in labour

'*For the first stage I began by keeping upright and walking round the delivery room; then during the contractions I leant slightly forward and held onto the end of the bed while my husband massaged my back. I moved my hips in circles during the contractions. I didn't find them at all painful, only uncomfortable.*'

With your body vertical, the descent of the baby is helped by the downward force of gravity. Some women like to stand up throughout labour – even for delivery. Others have remarked that holding on to a rope or pole and hanging minimises the pain (there are records of primitive women doing the same thing). It can be helpful to put your arms around the neck of another person and hang. The supporter should keep his or her shoulders down, bend the knees slightly and tighten the buttock muscles in order to carry your weight without getting an aching back. It is helpful to practise this.

Many women find it comforting to be held during the contractions and have a need for the close bodily contact of another person – often another woman. Some women prefer to be alone during labour with partner and midwife nearby in another room. Some like to stand, leaning forward on to the wall during contractions and squat in between them on a low stool.

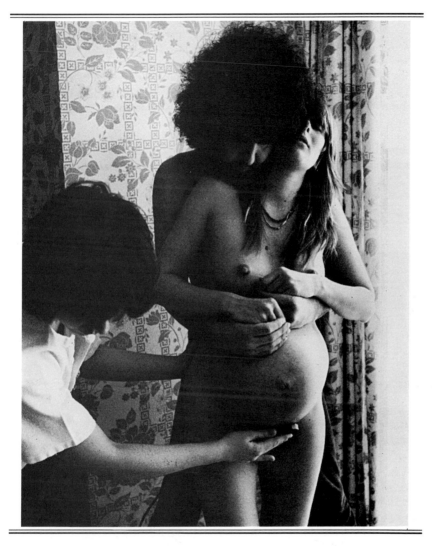

The midwife uses a handheld monitor to listen to the baby's heartbeat

'*Later in the afternoon my man and I went walking alone. I just wanted to hold him during the contractions. I felt such a strength from his energy. When I came into the house the contractions were very strong and I held Kurt round the neck and hung down. Until the final stage of my labour I had not related much to my man, finding I needed the soft quality of a woman but at the end it was wonderful to have his support, both mental and physical.*'

Squatting is the physiological position for labour and birth. Your pelvis is at its most open, gravity is helping and contractions are at their strongest. However, it is important not to tire yourself out and to rest completely in between contractions. Use the support of another person or a stool, a pile of books or a firm cushion to make yourself as comfortable as possible.

You may squat during contractions or in between them. Squatting is very useful at any stage of labour, particularly if you wish to speed things up. Some women find this the most comfortable posture.

Some women prefer to reserve squatting until the very end and to use other supported upright positions which are less tiring, such as kneeling forward over a bean-bag. Squatting during contractions will intensify them. In between, it will help to widen your pelvis and encourage the baby's descent.

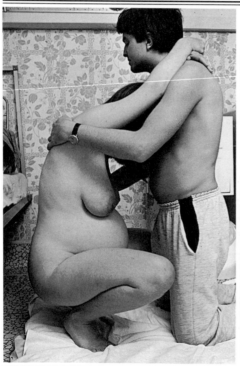 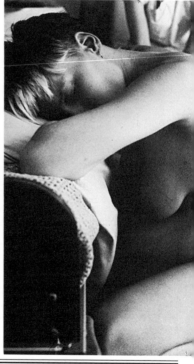

Supported squatting in labour   *Squatting leaning forward on bed*

'I continued to squat through contractions as this position seemed most natural and comfortable to me, especially spreading my knees as wide apart as I could and squirming from side to side, all the while trying to keep my breathing slow and deep, concentrating on breathing out.'

The sitting position

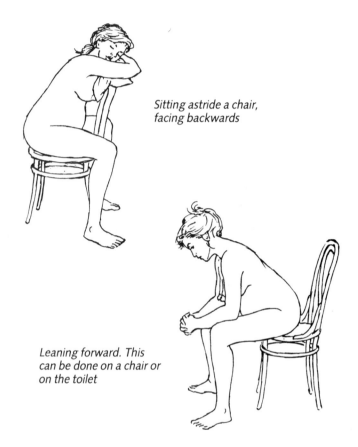

Sitting astride a chair, facing backwards

Leaning forward. This can be done on a chair or on the toilet

In these positions you have almost the same advantages as in squatting, and your trunk is supported. You can rest quite comfortably between contractions.

'I became absorbed by the contractions. I felt pain but not fear and trusted the process that was happening. I had the need to be on my own. I walked, knelt and squatted as the contractions increased. I found that the toilet seat was a very comfortable place because it supported me while leaving my pelvic floor free.'

The kneeling position is often used throughout labour, indeed most women find that, as labour intensifies and advances to the last part of the first stage (say, 7–10cm dilation), kneeling is the most comfortable. You may find it helpful to move your pelvis rhythmically during contractions, either rotating or rocking.

'I went on all fours where I found a gentle rocking movement eased the pain. My boyfriend rubbed the lower part of my back almost continuously.'

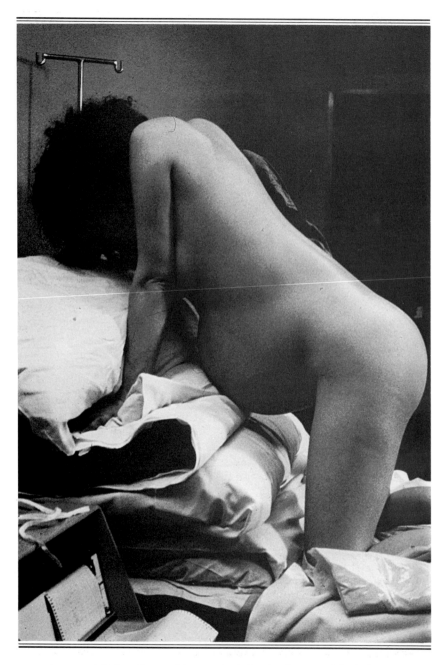

In an upright kneeling position gravity helps the descent of the baby

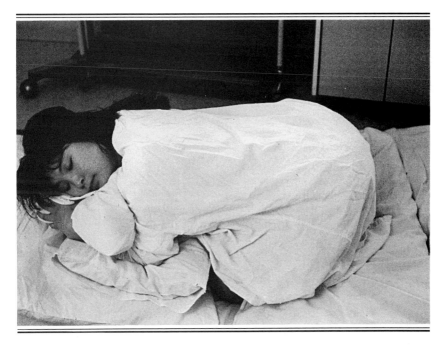

Resting in between contractions

The kneeling positions are very helpful if you have a 'backache labour' or if the baby is lying in a posterior position (see Chapter 10). Rhythmic rotation or spontaneous movement of the pelvis can help the baby to turn to the more usual anterior position.

You may prefer to kneel with your trunk upright or to lean forward on to a firm pile of cushions or piece of furniture. Make sure that the angle of your trunk is quite vertical to allow gravity to assist you.

'When the contractions became much stronger I moved to the bean-bag. I rested against this and rotated my hips. It really did help, in fact it seemed the most natural thing to do!'

If labour is progressing rapidly, you could use a more horizontal kneeling position if you wish to slow things down a little. The less vertical and more horizontal your body, the slower the contractions, as the downward force of gravity on the cervix lessens. In the case of a very sudden and fast birth, the knee-chest position will help to slow down the contractions and make them less overwhelming.

'All I knew was that I was going like the clappers and wanted to slow it down. I was kneeling on the floor so I put my head down on to the floor and my bottom up in the air.'

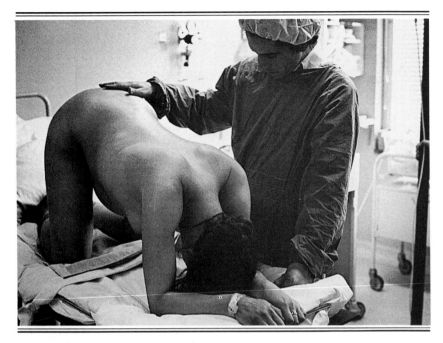

Kneeling head down is helpful during intense contractions

You will find that you can relax totally in between contractions in the kneeling position and the pain is more bearable. Use a foam pad in a pillow case or a folded blanket under your knees.

Kneeling is used in many religions as a position for prayer and helps one to enter a deeper level of consciousness, and to surrender to the powerful energy of the contractions within your body.

Half-kneeling and half-squatting is a good position to use combined with kneeling, and is easier than squatting. Change legs for each contraction and rock forwards and backwards towards your upper knee during contractions. This posture assists the dilation and may ease backache.

'I found the half-kneeling position comfortable, in fact it was during a strong contraction in the latter position that the waters broke and I found that a great relief.'

If you wish to lie down during the first stage, it is preferable to do so on your side, with your trunk well propped up by cushions and perhaps a pillow under one knee. Resting between contractions is important so be careful not to misinterpret the word 'Active' and exhaust yourself. Rather, find ways of relaxing and releasing in the action during contractions, and resting in between them.

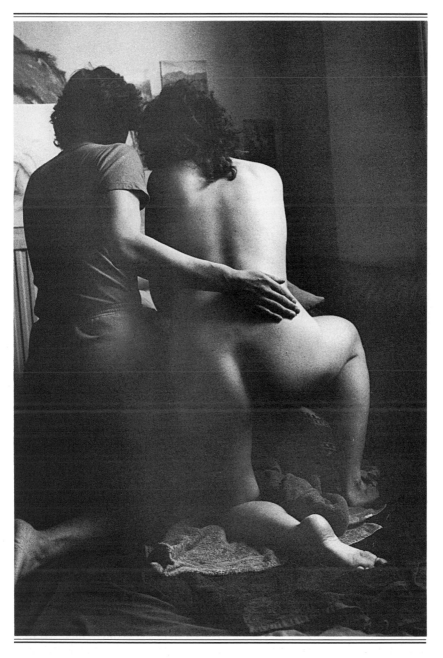

Half-kneeling, half-squatting during labour

Transition – the end of labour

I once heard a midwife explain to a woman in labour that the first stage was rather like climbing a high mountain and at the end of the steep incline one reaches a very difficult craggy bit. Although the top and the view down the other side is close at hand, one can lose sight of the end and fall into despair, struggling with these last difficult contractions.

This is an apt description of transition. It is like a bridge between the last dilating contractions and the beginning of the bearing down in the second stage. Transition can last for as little as a few seconds or as long as two or three hours or more. It is more common to have a long transition with a first birth.

Transition is a very sensitive time – while the final opening is taking place you are on the threshold of giving birth. Like the moment before orgasm, you will need to be without disturbance or distraction to let go to the involuntary impulses which will bring your baby to birth.

WHAT HAPPENS TO YOU

Your contractions are coming fast and furious with very short intervals between them. Your cervix is probably 8–9cm dilated, but that last centimetre may be very slow in disappearing. A common occurrence at this stage is what is known as an anterior lip, i.e. the front rim or lip of the cervix still needs to be taken up before the way is clear to bear down and push your baby out.

HOW YOU FEEL

This is not easy to describe!

Most women find this the most trying part of the labour. There you are, wide open and completely vulnerable. It is too late to take anything (and very unwise). You are not yet ready to bear down, although you may begin to feel the first urges. You may be feeling desperate, irritable and frightened at one moment and then suddenly blissful or ecstatic. At this stage you can feel that you have reached the end of your tether and may forget that you are about to give birth to a baby, and lose faith in everything. You are still feeling the final dilating contractions which are opening your womb to its widest, while the very different bearing down urges may be beginning. This can result in a feeling of confusion, of not knowing what is happening or where you are. In a while, when the expulsive contractions are established the confusion will pass.

The sensations you will be feeling will be very powerful. You may feel nauseous or trembly, your head may be hot while your feet may be cold. The important thing to remember is that it will pass and that the long haul of the first stage is almost over. Most women appear to be in a kind of trance at this stage of labour – in a very deep and open state of consciousness.

Transition

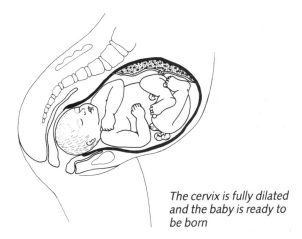

The cervix is fully dilated and the baby is ready to be born

'*I squatted or knelt on the mattress, supported on both sides by my friend and my husband, and I had a rather short, but extremely relaxed transition period. I believe I even slept for a spell.*'

'*This was the most difficult part as I didn't realise I was in transition and felt I wanted to push. I was worried as this seemed far too early to want to push. I knelt forward on the cushions. I found that eye contact with my husband was important at this stage. When I felt panic during transition my husband breathed with me to slow my breathing down. This immediately brought me back in control.*'

It is common to feel frightened during transition – after all, you are about to give birth and see your baby for the first time! Many women feel that they cannot do it or even that they may split apart or die. These fears are irrational and sometimes not even conscious. Michel Odent calls this 'physiological fear' and believes that this fear just before giving birth has a useful function in raising the level of adrenalin. He suggests that whereas in labour adrenalin could inhibit the work of the endorphin-like hormones, now it has a useful function in helping to trigger off the involuntary expulsive reflex of the second stage, which Michel calls 'the foetus ejection reflex'. He stresses the importance of not being overly reassuring or disturbing the mother at this stage. In his observations, if she is left more or less alone to experience this fear, a quick and efficient expulsive reflex usually follows (1–2).

You may feel very thirsty and want to drink a glass or two of water. This unusual thirst, together with the dilation of the pupils which is common in transition, are signs of an increase in adrenalin.

For some women, being completely alone in a darkened room can help to get through this stage, while others may need sensitive, non-intrusive support.

WHAT HAPPENS TO YOUR BABY

Your baby descends a little further into the pelvic canal. The uterus has been drawn up around the baby's head so that he or she is beginning to move out of the uterus ready to be born.

POSITIONS AND MOVEMENT FOR TRANSITION

Once again, follow your own instincts and use any position you have found helpful so far.

The kneeling position is the most popular at this stage. Use a good firm pile of cushions or else lean forward on to another person so that you can rest completely supported in the short breaks between contractions. Allow yourself to sink into a deep inner relaxation.

It is helpful to take sips of water, or to suck on a natural sponge – women often experience a primitive sucking reflex during labour. Bathe your face with a face cloth rinsed out in cold water to refresh yourself between contractions. You may like to sit back on your heels and stretch your arms up between contractions.

'*My mother-in-law gave me sips of warm water with a little honey added and washed my hands and face. Another thing which I found very comforting and refreshing during the whole labour, was to suck upon a wet sponge.*'

If you have a very long transition, try changing positions from time to time; sitting upright on the edge of the bed or on a chair, standing up, walking slowly or lying on your side well propped up by cushions. Many women find it helpful to sit on the toilet in transition.

KNEE-CHEST POSITION FOR AN ANTERIOR LIP

Although it is not usually necessary, your midwife may want to examine you internally at this stage to see if you are fully dilated. If she cannot feel the cervix at all you are ready to bear down and give birth to your baby. If, however, she can still feel a little rim of cervix in front of the baby's head, this is called an anterior lip. You may already be feeling the first urges to bear down, and may be advised to wait until the lip has gone. If the urge to bear down is irresistible the lip will probably move out of the way with your expulsive efforts.

It is not a good idea to resist the powerful bearing down urges so try the knee-chest position for a few contractions, with your head lower than your bottom.

This position brings the baby forward and reduces pressure on the cervix. Move your hips a little during contractions to assist the dilation. The lip will probably have gone after a few contractions. If the urge to bear down is very strong then try blowing out firmly when you have the urge, as if you are blowing out a candle three feet away. It is usually not necessary to stay in this position for longer than four or five contractions.

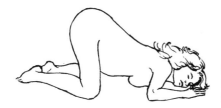

Knee chest position –
useful for slowing down
strong contractions

'Billie felt an anterior lip and I went into knee-chest position to counteract the strong pushing urge. Fortunately, after only a few contractions and blowing, it went and I got up.'

BREATHING FOR TRANSITION

Keep your deep breathing as usual, concentrating on the exhalation. If your breathing naturally becomes shallower then follow your own instincts. It will help you to be more relaxed if you focus your attention on the out-breath.

Most women need to shout out, moan, curse or make a lot of noise at this stage of the labour and find that it helps to relieve pain, whilst others need to be very quiet. It is most important that you should not be disturbed or distracted unnecessarily. Peace and quiet will help you to sink deeply inwards at this stage.

'The thing I found a tremendous help and relief was making a furious grunting, squealing noise at the height of each pain. It was a way of controlling myself both physically and mentally.'

'The contractions were very powerful and I began to feel extremely tired between them. I flopped forward on to two big cushions and felt as though I could sleep even for a few moments between contractions. The conservation of energy was simply wonderful. I didn't even speak when spoken to.'

The Second Stage of Labour

The second stage begins when the cervix is completely dilated and your baby's head has moved out of the uterus and into the birth canal. This stage ends with the perineum stage, or crowning, when your child is born.

WHAT HAPPENS TO YOUR CHILD

After full dilation of the cervix, your baby's head is free of the uterus and the contractions bring your child's head to the middle of the pelvic canal. At this point rotation begins as the head meets the pelvic floor. Descent continues, and there is further rotation as the head comes down under the pubic bone in front.

This may take time, and the rotation is usually complete before the back of the head reaches your vulva, although it may still be turning as it is born. Then the crown of your child's head appears, stretching your vaginal opening. With further contractions the child emerges as the face sweeps under your perineum. The body rotates, and first one shoulder and then the other emerges, until the child's body is rapidly expelled.

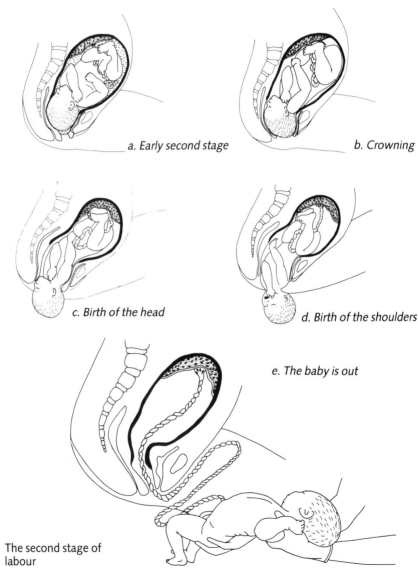

a. Early second stage

b. Crowning

c. Birth of the head

d. Birth of the shoulders

e. The baby is out

The second stage of labour

In passing through the pelvis, your child's head has been subjected to considerable pressure. That the descent is done without damage to the head is made possible by the softness of the bones themselves and because the edges of the skull bones are not yet fused, enabling them to overlap slightly. Your baby's head may seem slightly pointed in shape after birth due to this 'moulding' but will soon round out.

During the delivery, and for some time after, your child is still receiving oxygen from the placenta, through the umbilical cord. After the birth of the head the baby may take his first breath of air, but it will be a short while before full breathing is established.

Using upright positions for the second stage will help to ensure that your baby is getting as much oxygen as he needs and will minimise the pressure on his or her head.

WHAT HAPPENS TO YOU

You are fully dilated and ready to give birth to your baby. In the first part of the second stage, your uterus will begin to contract powerfully from above to push the baby down through the curved birth canal, under the pubic arch and on to the pelvic floor.

The expulsive contractions may start before you are fully dilated or they may begin 5–10 minutes or longer after dilation is complete. If you have a gap where nothing happens, make the most of it and rest in readiness for the birth. Occasionally this gap can last quite a long time but is followed by the expulsive reflex eventually.

If you have had a long transition your uterus may need to rest. There are great variations in the length of the second stage in different women, ranging between two and three minutes, and as many hours.

'My cervix was fully dilated but my body did not feel quite ready to push. It was resting, getting ready for the final stage. This lasted over an hour.'

HOW YOU FEEL

These contractions feel quite different from the previous ones. The intervals between them are generally longer. Even if you have felt very tired at the end of the first stage, a new rush of very powerful energy often comes to help you give birth to your baby. Women describe these contractions as huge tidal waves of sensation throughout the whole body. The expulsive reflex is completely involuntary and may come on quickly, or it may take a while before it starts.

'I wasn't sure what I was supposed to feel until suddenly I got a terrific urge to push which felt quite different to anything so far. With perfect timing, the doctor arrived. The second stage took half an hour but I had no sense of time. It seemed very quick to me.'

There is usually a tremendous urge to bear down, although this is not the case for all women. If you do not resist or run away from these feelings, but go along with them, they can be extremely enjoyable. The urge to bear down is very powerful and the muscular effort is often pleasurable. Pressure at this stage builds up enormously and any resistance to the expulsive effort causes discomfort and pain.

Try to allow the natural rhythm to lead you. Let your body be your guide and your uterus will take care of the rest.

'Nature took over. My whole body helped automatically and rhythmically in the enormous effort of pushing out a baby. I felt his head, shoulders and body being born.'

THE CROWNING

Your baby's head will extend backwards as it descends the birth canal. Finally, the crown of the baby's head will begin to show through your vagina. This is the right time to get into a suitable position for the birth of the baby. Feel his or her head with your hand as it descends. It is a memorable feeling and will help you to know exactly what is happening.

'I instinctively put my hand down to feel for the baby's head and there it was, crowning.'

To be born, your child will have to pass through your pelvic floor. In view of its action in childbirth, the pelvic floor can be regarded as consisting of two parts – the front, pubic part and the back, sacral part which is attached to your buttock bones, coccyx and sacrum. As your baby comes through, the pubic area is pulled inwards and the sacral part is pushed backwards, to make room for his head and body.

The pubic part has comparatively few voluntary muscles joining it to your pubic bones, whereas the sacral part has almost 90 per cent of all the pelvic floor muscles connected to it. This part of the pelvic floor is known as the perineum.

To be free to move backwards when the baby is born, the sacral area of the pelvic floor, or perineum, must be in a passive state of relaxation. The position of your body at this stage is all-important. If you are lying on your back, your sacrum is not free to move backwards, and the back sacral part of your pelvic floor is not in a passive relaxed state. This forces your child's head to press forward towards the bony sub-pubic arch, instead of backwards towards your sacrum and coccyx which are mobile and extendable. But if you are squatting, kneeling or standing, the position of your pelvis is altered and your sacrum and coccyx are extended back. Your back sacral area will be relaxed if your child's head presses against it, allowing as much give as possible.

The crowning ends with the birth of the baby. You may have one contraction when your baby's head is born and then a pause before the next contraction when the rest of the body emerges. Alternatively, the baby may be born in one contraction. Once the head is born, your baby will turn and first one shoulder and then the other will appear and finally the whole body will slip out.

HOW YOU FEEL

At this stage, the sensations one feels are very intense – a unique mixture of pain and ecstasy.

At the end of the crowning, when the head is about to be born and the perineal tissues stretch to their maximum, there can be a feeling of acute stretching and burning, similar to how it feels when you pull at the corners of your mouth with your fingers, mingled with the total body sensation of the contractions. However, as soon as the head, which is the widest part of the baby's body, is born, there is a tremendous feeling of relief. Sometimes, if the baby is broad shouldered, one can feel further stretching as first one shoulder and then the other is born, but as your baby's body slithers out into the world the sensations are usually very pleasurable and often described as totally orgasmic.

'That was the only pushing I did. The baby came out so gradually and easy without any pushing from me. I felt a burning sensation in my perineum as he was being born and, on checking, I didn't even have a tear.'

'I felt an incredible presence in the room and feelings were high. The pain was almost unbearable yet now the overpowering urge to bear down was there. It was one of the most powerful bodily sensations I think I have ever had and soon I saw her head in the mirror, a patch of thick black hair. With an extraordinary release of energy her head came out, but the energy to push was so strong that immediately after, her whole body shot out. The emotion was of the utmost release and joy and wonder and thankfulness. Words can not express that feeling at the moment of birth. I wanted to cry and shout for joy.'

BREATHING FOR THE SECOND STAGE

There is usually no need to control your breathing in the second stage of labour if you are in an upright, squatting or kneeling position.

Breathe deeply in the usual way as you feel the contraction coming on, concentrating on the out-breath and giving way to the powerful messages coming from inside your body. There is a distinctive birth cry which is natural and instinctive during the second stage, particularly as the baby is actually being born. It is unwise to resist these natural urges to cry out as they are nature's way of assisting you to give birth.

Do not tense up against the contractions of your uterus as this can be very painful. Just let yourself go and release your pelvic floor. Let your breath go and let the sound out as you allow your baby to be born. Women often say that when they screamed during the second stage, they felt no pain at all.

You will probably feel very powerful bearing-down urges and an uncontrollable desire to push downwards at the peak of the contraction, as your uterus presses down to expel your baby. Follow the natural urges of your body. Do not hold your breath for a long time as this diminishes the supply of oxygen going to you and your baby, at a time when it is critical that he should have enough.

At the crowning of your baby's head, try not to push too hard as this will lessen the chances of a perineal tear. Some women find it helpful to pant as the head is born, while others prefer to abandon themselves completely at this moment.

'I squatted on the bed supported by the midwife and my husband and felt my baby emerging. I put my arms under me and feeling the head I let out an unearthly primitive moan, letting the baby slide into my hand. She was warm, creamy, smoother and softer than anything I had ever touched.'

If the second stage is difficult – for instance, if you have a very large baby, an unusual presentation or a very slow second stage – you may find it helpful to bear down actively during the contraction. Wait until the contraction begins and then take in a good breath and, as you exhale, direct your energy downwards, pressing down inside with your diaphragm muscle, in exactly the same way as you would do to help yourself when defecating. It is not necessary to hold your breath. Sometimes lots of little pushes work better than one long one. Practise this gently in the squatting position in case you need to use it in labour.

Above all, in the second stage, keep in harmony with the rhythmic sensations you are feeling. Allow them to lead you, surrendering to what your body is telling you.

'During the 1½ hours of second stage, I was squatting on the floor almost the whole time, occasionally standing. I felt as comfortable as I could imagine being in labour and the position, being well supported, enabled me to control my breathing and work with the expulsive contractions as much as possible. I also had a really good view of the emerging head in a mirror propped up in the front of me. I gave birth to the baby in the same squatting position.'

POSITIONS FOR THE SECOND STAGE

Your posture makes all the difference to the length and efficiency of the second stage. You will make your child's descent easier if you use vertical, upright positions which allow gravity to help in the safe delivery of your child. Any standing, sitting, kneeling or squatting position is fine until the baby's head crowns. Then you need to get into a suitable position for the birth.

To understand the advantage of being upright . . .

TRY THIS

Squat down on your toes. Breathe in and tighten your pelvic floor, hold for a second and then let go slowly as you breathe out. Repeat several times.

Now try the same thing lying down in the reclining position with a pillow under your head. You will probably find that, in this position, the movement of your perineum is much weaker and more effort is needed on your part to let go of the pelvic floor muscles.

Try it again squatting and compare the difference when gravity helps the pelvic floor to relax.

The fit between your child's head and your pelvis is so exact that the smallest increase in the size of your pelvis is significant.

TRY THIS

Squat down on your toes and spread your knees apart. Close your eyes and be aware of the opening of your pelvis. In fact, it is open at its widest in this position and your sacrum and coccyx are free to move if your child is passing through your pelvic outlet.

Now try the semi-reclining position. Place your hand under your back and feel how the whole weight of your body, your uterus and baby is lying on your sacrum which is closed to its maximum, in this position. Research suggests that you are losing a significant percentage (up to one third) of the possible opening.

The weight of your uterus also presses down on the large internal blood vessels in your abdomen in a reclining position, which reduces the supply of oxygen going to your baby and is likely to induce foetal distress. Your uterus tilts forward when it contracts. In the semi-reclining position it must work against the downward force of gravity. This will make contractions more painful and less effective.

'On one occasion I was lying on my back to enable Jane to examine me. Unfortunately I had a contraction whilst in this position. It was extremely painful and I would not like to repeat that experience.'

Your coccyx is designed to move out of the way as your baby's head descends to make more room – all the more reason not to sit on it! It can also lead to dislocation of the coccyx which can be extremely painful for months after the birth.

These are some of the reasons why women who have the freedom to choose their own positions for delivery, rarely choose the semi-reclining one, much less to lie down on their backs. (For instance, in one year at Pithiviers, only two out of one thousand women chose to lie down.)

Each position has certain advantages. You will find out instinctively which position is best for you at the time. Try them out with your partner in the weeks before the birth so your body will know all the possibilities. Also, sometimes, the room and circumstances in which you give birth will dictate the position you choose. Ideally, the room should contain little furniture so that you can freely discover the right posture. However, it is possible to use natural birth positions either on a bed or on the floor. (See Chapter 10.)

Unless the second stage is very short, it is likely that you will change positions – standing and squatting, or squatting and kneeling, or kneeling and sitting up – as your baby descends. It is helpful to have two people nearby to help support you.

Sitting on the toilet may be helpful as the baby descends, but once the head crowns and you feel the baby is coming, it is time to get into a supported squat.

Many women make the mistake of starting to squat too early. Any upright position will do until the head of the baby crowns and then it is time to use the birth position. If the second stage is very rapid, you will probably feel like being on all-fours and you can remain there for the birth.

1   SUPPORTED SQUATTING

The standing, supported squat makes optimum use of gravity and is the most efficient position for the rapid descent of the baby.

You stand or walk in between contractions but as the contraction comes on, your knees will bend and you will feel the need to hold on to something, or someone can support you from behind while you let go of your weight and surrender to the force of the contraction.

After the contraction passes you move freely until the next one, when you are supported again.

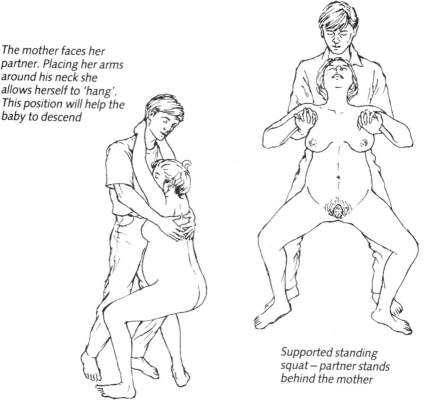

The mother faces her partner. Placing her arms around his neck she allows herself to 'hang'. This position will help the baby to descend

Supported standing squat – partner stands behind the mother

Tips for the supporter
Place your feet 2–3 feet apart. It is best to be without socks and shoes. Bend your knees and strengthen the muscles of the thighs and buttocks, leaning back just a little so that her weight is carried against your pelvis. Keep your back straight and resist the temptation to bend forward as this will put strain on your lower back. Keep your arms and shoulders relaxed so that the supporting strength is coming from your thighs while your upper body remains more or less free from tension.

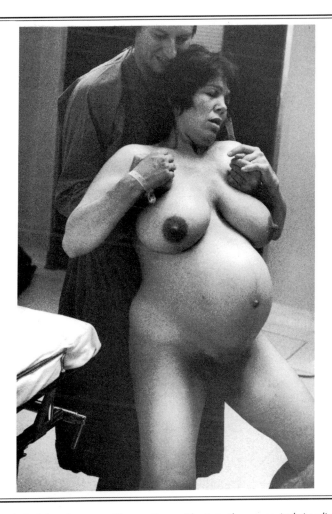

The baby's head crowns. The mother settles into the supported standing squat ready for the birth

Keep your knees bent and ground yourself by breathing deeply. Try exhaling 'through the soles of your feet', towards the floor to ground and relax yourself.

This should become easy with a little practice, and once you have the dynamics right even a small person can support a large and heavy woman with no strain or effort. If you have a weak back or any spinal problems, it is best to use a chair.

Once your feet and lower body are in position, you are ready to take your partner's weight.

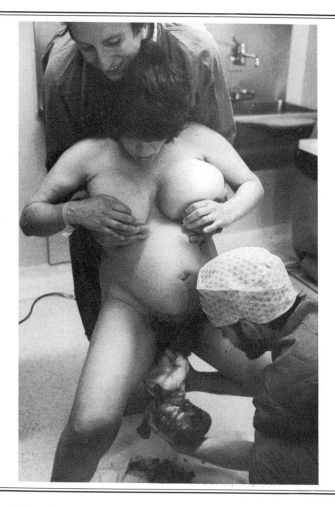

The baby is born in one contraction

Keeping your shoulders and upper arms relaxed, pass your hands under her arms with the palms uppermost. She can put her hands on top of yours, placing the palms together, and link her fingers with yours. Then relax together and let her hold on to you, rather than vice versa. Keep your arms and hands as relaxed as possible. It is a good idea to place a bean-bag behind your legs as your partner might drop down very low as the baby is being born and you could then squat on the bean-bag and she can squat between your legs.

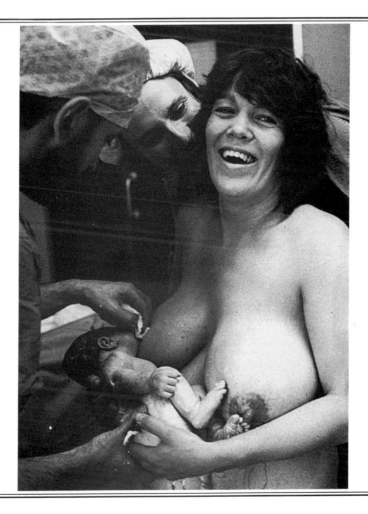

Moments after the birth

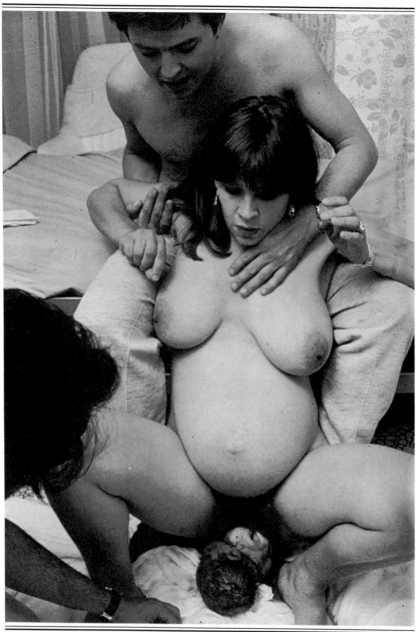

The baby emerges. The father sits on the edge of the bed and supports the mother as the baby is born ·

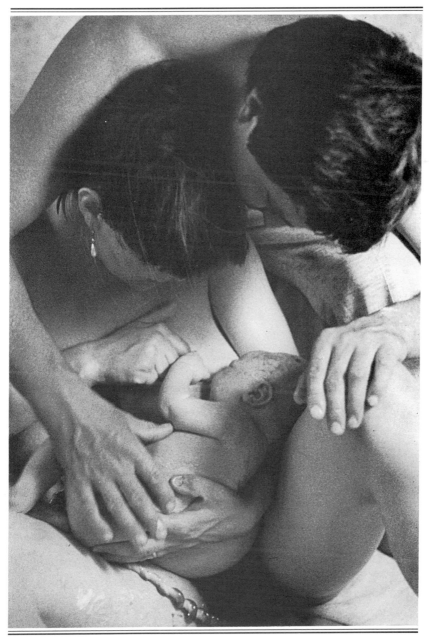

The mother and father welcome their newborn baby. The placenta is still attached and the cord has not yet been cut

Alternative hand position

It may be more comfortable to hold the hands palm to palm without linking the fingers or, alternatively, the mother could make fists with her thumbs up and her supporter can grasp her thumbs.

Tips for the mother

Once you have the position right, then relax completely against your partner's body. Allow yourself to be heavy as you go down into a squat but keep your feet flat, if possible, so that they carry some of your weight. Let go of any tension in your neck and rest your head back against your partner's body. Then, with legs apart and heavy pelvis, let go to the powerful contractions which bring the baby to birth.

Once the baby is born, the midwife could place it safely down in front of you, on an absorbent towel, then sit down to welcome your baby!

Tips for the midwife

The position for delivery should only be assumed once the baby's head is crowning.

Lifting the mother up from the kneeling position into a supported standing squat when the baby's head crowns

Taking her time the mother stands up. As she does so her partner moves back a little and adopts the standing position for a supported squat

The partner takes hold of the mother's thumbs. She rises slowly into an upright kneeling position

The partner stands over the mother and passes his hands under her arms in between contractions

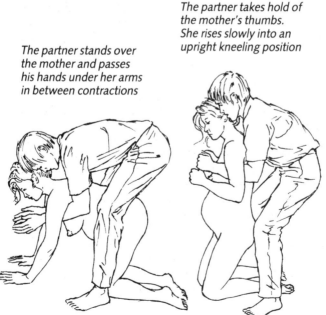
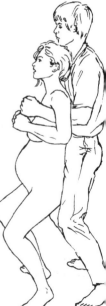

A clean sheet covered with an absorbent towel or disposable paper pad can be placed between the mother's legs ready to receive the baby. There is usually no need to guard the perineum as the baby will probably be born quite quickly but, if the final stage is slow, a warm compress held against the perineum will help to prevent tearing and will be soothing for the mother.

Usually the mother does best without any instructions at all so that she can simply surrender to her body's urges and cry out as the baby is being born. Some women prefer some sensitive guidance at this point. It is very important to wait for the expulsive reflex to come on spontaneously, without disturbing the mother or giving her unnecessary instructions. In an upright position it is not generally necessary to encourage the mother to 'push' but rather to enable her to 'let go' without inhibition.

A firm foam mat about 2 inches thick which is covered with a washable cover is useful to place on the floor and the baby can be placed face-down (on his belly) on an absorbent towel (or a non-slip, light, washable yoga mat) for a few minutes until the mother is ready for the first contact. In this way the fluids will drain naturally with the help of gravity, and suction is very rarely needed. The mother should remain sitting upright in the third stage to facilitate first contact and the separation of the placenta. Syntometrine is not needed to facilitate the third stage unless there is excessive bleeding.

Advantages
In this position the pelvis is wide open and the verticality makes for maximum help from gravity. The upward force of the supporter's body acts as a counterbalance to the downward force of the contractions.

The second stage tends to be quickest in this posture, the baby usually comes out in one contraction after the crowning. This is a great advantage if the second stage has been long or difficult, or when there is a difficult presentation (e.g. posterior or breech), a big baby or if there is any suspicion of distress (which is less likely if the labour has been active).

The simplicity of this position allows the mother great freedom to act instinctively – to surrender to her natural urges. After the birth, the simple upright sitting position facilitates an ideal bonding of mother and child, as anyone will know who has tried to put a baby to the breast while lying back.

> '*With the first urges to bear down I searched for a posture to help me do so. The best one was with my husband holding me up from the back with his arms passing under mine and locked in front of me while I just let myself hang loose. It was not only a comfortable position for me but one where the sheer contact with his physical strength revived my now tired body, and it also gave us both a sense of bonding. The bearing down happened on its own and within just four pushes our baby was out: a beautiful, slippery, gurgly little girl.*'

A bath of warm water can be brought for the infant and placed between the mother's legs so that she can bathe her baby before the placenta is delivered or the umbilical cord is cut. Alternatively, mother and baby could bathe together in the bathtub a little later after the placenta is delivered or not at all.

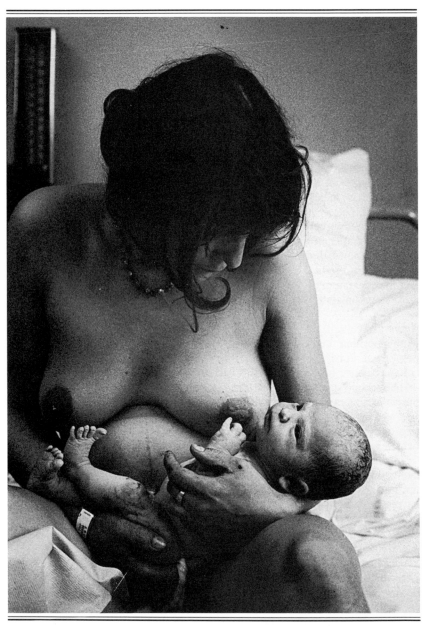

The mother sits upright on a hospital delivery bed moments after an active birth. In this position she enjoys perfect contact with her baby. The baby opens his eyes and first eye contact takes place

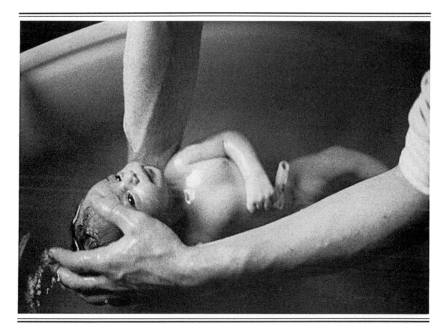

The baby being bathed soon after birth

The loving feelings of the mother in this first contact between her and her baby – skin to skin and eye to eye – encourage the production of natural hormones, which stimulate the separation of the placenta and the contraction of the uterus in the third stage.

'He stared intently at me and then started to suck at my breast. The cord was left attaching us until it stopped pulsing and was white. There was no feeling of separation, only continuation and deep joy and contentment. Everything felt right and I felt wonderful, not at all tired.'

2 SUPPORTED SQUATTING WITH TWO PEOPLE

This position may be ideal for the woman who can squat easily or has practised squatting throughout her pregnancy. The pelvis is open at its widest and gravity helps the baby to descend. During the contraction the mother squats down on the ground and her two supporters kneel on either side of her placing one knee just under her buttocks. She can then put one arm around the shoulders of each supporter who, in turn, can put one arm each around her back. Between contractions she can stand up or kneel forward.

It is important that the supporters are comfortable kneeling and it helps to place a cushion between the calves and buttocks or under the knees.

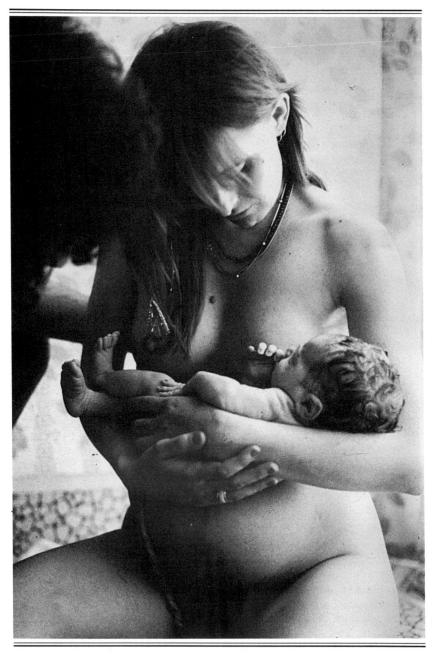

Kneeling, upright, the mother cradles her newborn baby in her arms

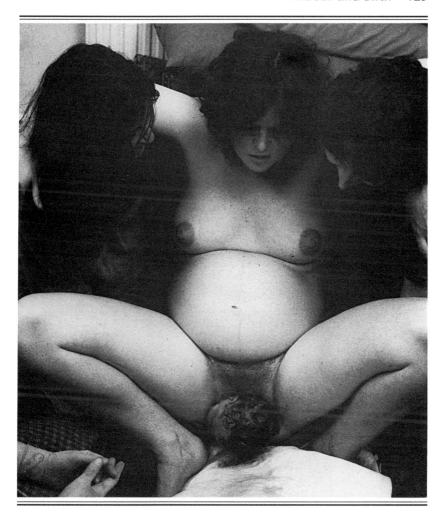

Supported squatting with two people. The midwife waits for the baby to emerge with the next contraction

Advantages

In this position the mother is free to use her hands and to look down and watch her baby being born in a completely relaxed, supported squat. Many women find it very helpful to use their own hands to feel the baby's head descending and to help ease the perineal tissues and deliver the baby as it is born. Some women have a strong instinct to do this themselves.

It is easy to stand up or kneel forward on to hands and knees from this position.

Nature has intended this position for birth because, in this full squatting position, the baby, unassisted, will slip out between the mother's legs and land safely in front of her, face downwards. She can then lift up the baby herself. This is also the safest position for the fluids to drain from the mother.

After the birth, the mother can sit down on the floor in an upright sitting position. It is much easier for the mother to handle the baby if she is upright and for the baby to find the breast.

'For the second stage I turned and proceeded to squat, standing up in between contractions to stretch the legs. All things considered, I felt marvellous – confident, in control – during this stage which lasted about three-quarters of an hour. The obstetrician, by turning his head for a moment, missed the actual birth. Lara literally sailed out – a totally solo performance – and exercised her vocal cords immediately!'

3   SUPPORTED SQUATTING USING A CHAIR

Here, the supporter sits on a chair or on the edge of a bed and the mother squats with her body cradled between his legs and uses his knees for support. Many women find this most enjoyable and comforting, as well as comfortable.

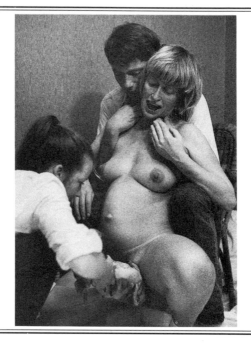

Supported squatting with the partner sitting on a chair. The mother cries out freely as the baby is born

It is best for the supporter to use a firm chair and to sit well forward on the edge so that the mother can rest against his body. This position is ideal if the supporting partner has a weak back.

'*I squatted between Ron's knees as he sat on a chair and I supported myself on his thighs with my elbows, resting my back in his lap.*

'*We looked in the mirror to see our baby's head emerging, then before the midwife could put her gloves on, all of him was born and he was placed in my arms to suckle.*'

4   KNEELING OR ALL-FOURS POSITION

You simply kneel forward on to your hands and knees or on to a pile of cushions with your knees apart.

This position comes very naturally and is often used by women in traditional birth practice. It is ideal if the labour and second stage are very fast as you will have more control, and the baby will descend a little more slowly. It can also be very useful if the baby is in a posterior presentation as it relieves pressure on the back and you can move your hips gently to help the baby rotate as it descends. Mothers say that this is a very simple and easy way to give birth. In between contractions you can kneel upright and stretch your arms if you want to.

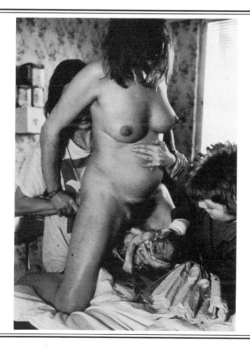

Kneeling upright the baby is born on the hospital delivery bed

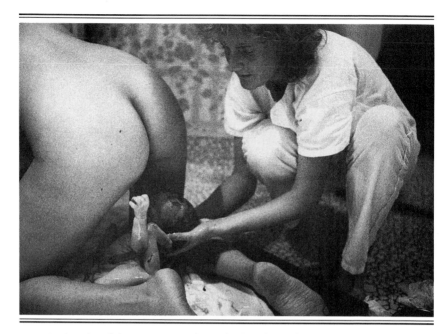

Birth in the all fours position. The midwife is dressed comfortably so that she too can be active!

Once the baby is born and is received by the midwife, she can pass the baby through your legs and place it face down in front of you. You can then sit back on your heels or upright to see and lift up your baby.

Some mothers instinctively turn over after delivery in a kneeling position. The midwife can then pass the baby to the mother under one knee as she turns. Often mothers deliver in a more upright kneeling position with one knee up. This position can be useful if the mother wishes to deliver the baby herself.

In the case of a very fast and unexpected second stage, use the knee-chest position to slow down and gain control (see page 110).

'When the second stage began I knelt upright and held on to the top of the bed to push. It took no more than half an hour to push the baby out. I gave birth on all-fours then, without having the cord cut, I turned over and was given the baby. Wonderful! Because I was kneeling and very much in control of how fast the baby was being born, I didn't tear and so was able to walk around quite comfortably shortly after delivery.'

Birth in the kneeling
position

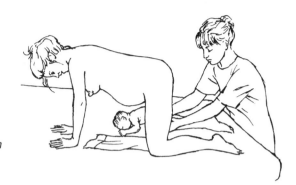

*The baby is passed
through the mother's
knees after birth and
placed face down on an
absorbent towel*

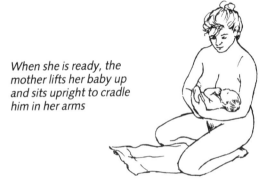

*When she is ready, the
mother lifts her baby up
and sits upright to cradle
him in her arms*

5 SIDE LYING

This can sometimes be a useful position for delivery. The sacrum is free to
move but gravity will not be used to full advantage so this posture would not be
sensible if the second stage was slow. However, when the baby is descending
without difficulty, you may be comfortable like this.

Lie on your side with your trunk well propped up by pillows and hook one
arm under your knee to support your leg as the baby is born.

After the birth, sit upright to hold and put your baby to the breast.

*'For me, the right position was simply the one which felt right at the time. This was
lying on my left side with my knee drawn to my chest and my hands drawing the
opening wider and, at the same time, being able to have contact with the emerging
head. In this way I was able to actively open my perineum with its delicate muscles
and give a little tactile help.'*

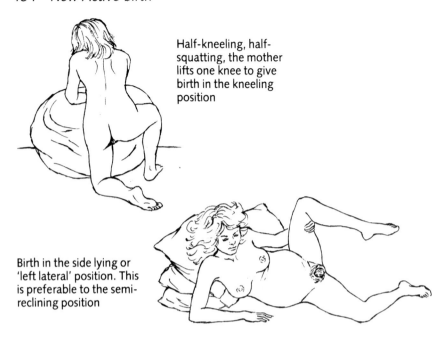

Half-kneeling, half-squatting, the mother lifts one knee to give birth in the kneeling position

Birth in the side lying or 'left lateral' position. This is preferable to the semi-reclining position

THE BABY IMMEDIATELY AFTER BIRTH

As he is born, and immediately after birth, your baby may be a slightly blue or greyish colour. This is perfectly normal and as soon as breathing starts the body will become the normal pink colour.

The baby will be very slippery and moist, perhaps covered in some blood and a white creamy substance which looks rather like butter and is called vernix. This is important to the baby and should not be washed off as it contains nourishing substances which are absorbed by the baby's body and also protects the baby from the change in temperature from your body to the room. Within a few hours, this will be absorbed by the skin.

The baby may be a little wrinkled too, but after some time the body becomes soft and round. Some babies also have fine hairs growing on their ears or other parts of the body at birth; these will fall out in the early weeks. The baby's head at this age is quite large in proportion to the rest of the body and could be a little pointed or 'moulded' from the birth, and the genitals are usually a little enlarged as well.

Your baby's eyes will open very soon after the birth – perhaps even before the whole body emerges – and will be awake and looking for you! All the baby's senses are acutely sensitive and alive at this stage. The skin, ears and eyes and mouth are all receptive to any stimulation. For this first hour or two after birth, the baby will be extremely alert – more so than in the hours and days to come – as she or he experiences the world, the atmosphere, breathing and sight for the first time. The lungs and digestive system begin to work independently as the baby breathes air and sucks colostrum from your breasts.

The baby will need to keep close to you, to the familiar sound of your heartbeat and the warmth of your body, in the early hours, days and weeks after birth.

The Third Stage of Labour

After the birth your baby will be in your arms. The rush of emotion will cause the secretion of hormones in your body which, after a while, will cause your uterus to contract and the placenta to separate from the wall of the uterus. Nature has designed the process to take place quite automatically. As your baby comes into contact with the breast or sucks on the nipple, this causes the secretion of hormones which cause the uterus to contract strongly.

Meanwhile, your baby begins to breathe independently through the lungs and, after 10 to 15 minutes (if not sooner), breathing will be fully established and the umbilical cord will have stopped pulsating. The placenta and cord continue functioning until breathing is fully established to guarantee the baby a supply of oxygen and a means of getting rid of carbon dioxide. Particularly in the case of distress or a complication, this supply of oxygen is a natural insurance that the baby will receive sufficient oxygen until he or she is capable of breathing independently.

It is extremely dangerous for a newborn baby to be deprived of oxygen and this can cause brain damage. It is equally dangerous for the baby to have no means of breathing out carbon dioxide. If the baby is still receiving oxygen from the placenta (if the umbilical cord is not cut prematurely) this is far less likely to occur.

A midwife once told me a story of an unusual situation in a rural area where there was no back-up and the baby was breathing irregularly for an hour and a half. She left the cord attached and also gave the baby some oxygen occasionally until the breathing was regular. She observed that the cord continued to function for one and a half hours and then finally stopped pulsating when the baby no longer needed to breathe through the placenta. The placenta then separated and was delivered and the baby was in perfect condition.

After the cord has stopped pulsating it becomes completely flaccid and clamps itself spontaneously. It is then appropriate to cut the cord and to separate the baby from the placenta. Many parents enjoy cutting the cord themselves – a ritual of separation which can be very satisfying. The cord can be cut after it stops pulsating or after the placenta is delivered at the very end.

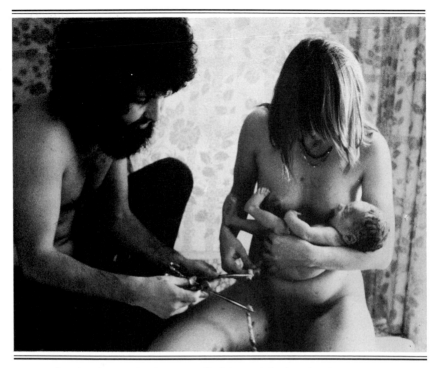

After the placenta has been expelled the umbilical cord is clamped and then the father cuts it

The third stage should not be rushed. Artificial stimulants (Ergometrine or Syntometrine) which induce contractions of the uterus, are not generally necessary after Active Birth if the normal bonding situation has occurred and if the mother has given birth in an upright position. These are best used in situations where the mother has been lying down during labour and has had an epidural or other anaesthetic or form of intervention which reduces the ability of the uterus to contract spontaneously, in the unusual case of excessive bleeding, or when mother and baby are separated at birth and the normal hormonal secretion is disturbed. Syntometrine is still given routinely in most hospitals. You may need to discuss this with your birth attendants in advance. Giving birth actively diminishes the risk of postpartum haemorrhage. Syntometrine has certain risks which make it inadvisable as routine practice when labour and birth have been normal and spontaneous (see page 187).

After the birth, the suckling of the baby at the breast will stimulate the uterus to contract and expel the placenta. This usually occurs in the first hour after birth but can sometimes take longer. There is no need to hurry the process unless there is excessive bleeding.

You will feel the contractions coming on and could then squat in order to allow the uterus to expel the afterbirth. It is approximately one-third the size of the baby and, unlike the baby, has no bones and is much easier to deliver. The sensations women feel as the placenta comes out are very enjoyable – it is like ending on a pleasant and healing note.

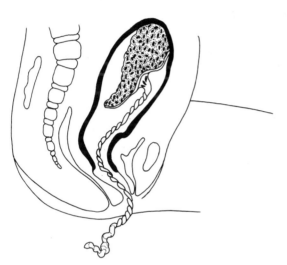

Separation of the placenta

'The placenta was born half an hour later. I simply squatted over a dish and with one gentle push out it came!'
If the third stage is spontaneous there is a far less likelihood of any complication occurring. This is one of the main reasons why cord-traction (where the midwife pulls on the cord to deliver the placenta) is not usually advisable. Although it won't hurt, it robs you of the orgasmic pleasure of delivering the placenta spontaneously, and there is more risk of a fragment of placenta being left behind, which could cause an infection.

Remember to have a look at the placenta if you want to. Hospitals usually donate placentas to cosmetic factories which use the valuable hormones to make their products.

In some societies, extensive rituals surround the disposal of the afterbirth because it is often regarded as having been part of the baby in the womb, and as having magical properties. Many animals eat the placenta – the hormones it contains help the uterus to contract and return to normal. Now and then, women do the same thing (some cooking it into a stew with wine and mushrooms). Recent experiments have revealed that putting even one piece of raw placenta to the lips of the mother after birth causes the uterus to contract and can stop haemorrhages. Other people like to bury the placenta under a favourite tree (although the hospital staff will find this unusual), and some couples take it home in a plastic bag for burial.

After the birth your doctor will examine your vagina and perineum to see if you have torn and if any stitching up is needed. If this is the case, the doctor will give you a local anaesthetic to prevent you feeling any pain and then stitch up the tear. If you do need stitching you can, if you wish, continue to hold your baby while this is being done. It is advisable to use local anaesthesia as there is no danger to the baby and the stitching can be very painful without it. Even for one stitch it is worth the anaesthetic! It is not necessary to use foot stirrups if the anaesthesia is well administered as you should not feel anything. Soothing, antiseptic herbal baths will speed up the healing of tears or episiotomies (see page 196).

Your baby will also be examined to ensure perfect health and this too can be done while still in your arms, if you wish. Although labour is over, the third stage is a very important time for you, your partner and your baby. Your baby is at its most alert. You will be, in a sense, meeting each other for the first time, looking into each others' eyes and sharing your first hours together. A few hours later your baby will fall asleep and will be sleepy or feeding most of the time in the next week or so.

It is now widely recognised that you need to take your time together, to integrate and share your feelings, to celebrate the arrival of a new person to your family, and this bonding is an essential part of your new relationship with each other. Most of the procedures which need to be done, such as stitching and the detailed examination of the baby, can wait for an hour or so.

Try to spend a few hours together alone immediately after the birth if you are in hospital, and if you are at home this is the appropriate time for the whole family to be together. If complications at birth make this impossible then take the very first opportunity to be alone together in just the same way.

'He lay on me for an hour and a half, while we talked quietly, my husband and I thoroughly involved in getting to know our new little son. That night we were never separated. He lay calmly looking all around him with a quiet awareness before at last falling asleep. For me those hours will never be forgotten.'

7 | Water Birth

So far we have considered the effect of gravity on the normal physiology of the birth process, and how you can position your body in harmony with your own instincts and the downward gravitational force of the earth. We have observed the disadvantages of defying gravity if you were to lie back or remain immobile in the semi-reclining position.

When you enter a pool of warm water in labour, the buoyancy of the water reduces the effect of gravity, allowing you to float freely or change positions, more or less weightless. Many women feel attracted to water in labour, and find that immersion in a warm pool is a helpful way to relax and surrender to the involuntary forces at work in their bodies and to ease the pain and discomfort of strong contractions. Some women deliberately choose to remain in the pool during the second stage and to give birth under water. The value of using warm water during labour and birth is increasingly being recognised and will hopefully become a more popular option in the coming decades, so that many more women will have a pool available for their use in the birthing environment.

The History of Water Birth

Water is our original element. In the first nine months in the womb the foetus develops in the aquatic environment of the amniotic fluid. Like a miniature sea, the waters of the womb provide the ideal medium for the growing baby, protecting him or her from shock or injury. Bathing in water continues to play an important role throughout child and adult life as a way to relax and relieve tension. Water is used therapeutically for hydrotherapy and also for purification or sanctification in religious rituals all over the world.

In the last few decades there has been increasing interest in the use of water during pregnancy, birth and infancy. Combined with yoga, swimming in pregnancy is an ideal way to exercise. Free from the effects of gravity, the mother can enjoy a pleasant and relieving feeling of lightness as well as greater ease of movement, enhancing cardio-vascular fitness. Midwives have known for years that a warm bath can relax a mother and encourage the progress of her labour. However, the idea of a woman entering a pool of water deep enough to be fully immersed and the possibility of actually giving birth under water, was

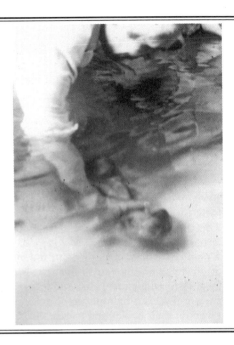

Michel Odent lifts a baby born in water from the bottom of the birth pool at Pithiviers

first explored fully by the Soviet researcher Igor Tjarkovsky in the 1960s, although his work was preceded by the work of several other Russian researchers (1,2,3). Later on in the same decade, the French obstetrician Frederick Leboyer introduced the idea of bathing newborn babies in warm water immediately after they had been born, to help them to acclimatise gradually and successfully to life outside their mother's womb.

Giving birth in water appeals to many parents as a way to ease the trauma of birth for their babies and to ensure a gentle transition from the protected watery world of the womb to the field of gravity on land, in infancy. It is estimated that throughout the world approximately 3000 babies have been born in water.

Another pioneer of water birth is Michel Odent, who first thought of using warm water as a way to ease pain during labour. He installed a simple inflatable pool adjoining the 'primitive' birthing room at the General Hospital in Pithiviers, France, in 1977, and by 1983 thousands of women had used the pool during labour and 100 of them had given birth under water (4). Odent emphasises that in his view the goal is not necessarily to give birth under water, but that the pool is offered as a possibility for those women who are attracted to use it. The warm water is a tool to help facilitate the labour and, while it is possible that the baby will be born under water, in his experience most women prefer to get out for the second stage.

Odent discovered that the pool was especially useful for women who were having long and painful labours (particularly backache) and who were having difficulty progressing beyond 5cms dilation. After entering the pool, they would dim the lights and usually the warm water would help the mother to reach full dilation within a couple of hours.

When the mother gave birth in the water, Odent observed that being in the pool seemed to enhance the first contact between mother and baby and that there were no special risks attached either to labour or birth under water (5). In the *Lancet*, Odent says, 'It should be possible for any conventional hospital to have a pool situated close to the birthing room and operating theatre . . . immersion in warm water is an efficient, easy and economical way to reduce the use of drugs and the rate of intervention in parturition'.

In the 1980s, the use of water pools has spread and there are many groups of people who have had similarly encouraging results, notably in the U.K., North America, Belgium, Scandinavia, Australia and New Zealand (6).

Using Water for Labour and Birth

It is generally thought that the best time to enter the pool is midway through labour at about 5cms dilation when the contractions are becoming very intense. (It has been observed that if a woman enters the pool in the early part of labour this can sometimes prolong labour and slow down contractions.) While this is a useful guideline, it may not apply to every woman and should not be used as a rule of thumb. If you feel an irresistable urge to enter the water this should not be denied. At the same time it is helpful to darken the room and to maintain a calm and peaceful atmosphere with attendants reduced to only those who are essentially needed. It is wise to listen to the foetal heart just before entering the pool and this can be repeated if necessary from time to time with a small hand-held ultrasound heart monitor (doptone) or a traditional obstetric stethoscope. (You will need to sit up on the edge of the pool as the transducer cannot be held under water, although some midwives report using a waterproof plastic bag to cover the transducer. However, it would certainly be ruined if wet accidentally.)

In the warm water, you can relax and let go, breathing calmly and deeply through the contractions, moving and changing positions to make yourself comfortable. It is possible to kneel over the edge, to squat, to semi-sit or to float as you please and, from time to time, you may enjoy immersing your whole body including your head under the water for short periods. You will find that the water allows you to enjoy the sensual pleasure of your body and to sink into the altered or expanded state of consciousness that naturally envelopes you as your womb opens up with each contraction. You will become less aware of what is happening around you and more able to surrender deeply to the instinctive and primitive urges of your body. Usually, once you have had a chance to relax in the water, labour progresses quite rapidly, and most women find that their perception of pain changes and it becomes much easier to accept the intensity of the contractions. It occasionally happens that contractions slow down and become less intense and if this situation persists, it is best to leave the pool and make use of gravity. After moving around for a while outside the pool and using upright resting positions, rhythmic contractions should soon build up again and labour will probably re-establish. It is important that the water temperature is comfortable, but not too warm.

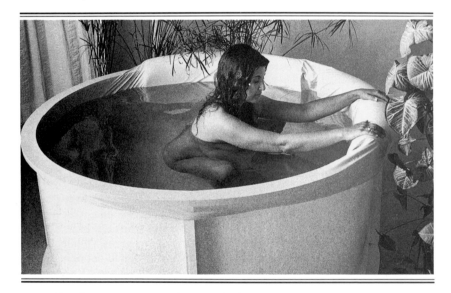

Kneeling or squatting in the water birth pool during strong labour helps to relieve pain and enhances contractions

When you reach full dilation you may wish to leave the pool. Should your membranes rupture there is no need to leave or change the water as the amniotic fluid and blood from a 'show' are sterile. Michel Odent reported in the *Lancet*, 'We had no infectious complications, even where the membranes were already broken.' There is no evidence of increased infection in any other centre where water births take place, in fact, it is considered that the use of a water pool might reduce the risk of infection, especially in a hospital where infection from 'foreign' bacteria in the air is more likely.

A water pool may also increase your sense of privacy in the hospital environment, giving you a space of your own to relax and feel safe in, where you can be less aware of what is going on around you. The immersion in warm water tends to lower high blood pressure caused by anxiety and certainly reduces pain (7). This is due to the loss of the effects of gravity and is also thought to be due to a fall in the catecholamine production (i.e. stress hormones like adrenaline), and an increase in the secretion of endomorphines (hormones which are natural relaxants and painkillers) caused by the warmth of the water.

Many hospitals and midwives who are apprehensive about the actual birth taking place under water, are open to the use of a water pool for labour. The provision of a pool for the latter part of the first stage is a completely safe and harmless way to facilitate your labour, and provides a risk-free alternative to medications or epidurals.

If a pool is not available any access to water will be helpful. It is possible, for example, to kneel in an ordinary bathtub with an attendant sponging warm water soothingly over your back. Try to make the water as deep as possible and comfortably warm. Alternatively, standing or squatting in the shower with the warm water running down your back or even sponging and splashing yourself with water from the hand basin will help you. Sometimes just the sound of a tap running can stimulate contractions and help you to let go of inhibitions. Warm or cold compresses, Evian sprays and hot-water bottles, ice or a natural sponge rinsed out in cold water, are all tried and tested labour aids.

GIVING BIRTH UNDER WATER

Labour might progress so quickly that there is no time to leave the pool and your baby is simply born into the water. Perhaps you will choose to stay in the water deliberately for the birth or, on the other hand, you may well feel like getting out. It is impossible to predict ahead of time whether your baby will be born in the water or not. Sometimes it is wise or necessary to leave the pool and take advantage of the help of gravity or a cooler atmosphere, to facilitate the second stage.

Reasons for leaving the pool might be:
• The mother feeling that she wants to leave the water.
• A prolonged second stage.
• Signs of possible foetal distress i.e. meconium released into the water.
• A breech birth (although some maintain that the warmth of the water might reduce the risk of the baby 'breathing' and hence the placenta separating, before the head emerges because it is not stimulated by the cooler temperature of the atmosphere on the skin. This has not been generally practised. Given the increased risk of a breech birth, it is wiser to make optimal use of gravity in the standing squat position. Michel Odent writes in the *Lancet* 'our strategy is to use the first stage as a test before deciding on either a vaginal delivery or a Caesarian section: in these cases we prefer not to interfere with drugs or with a bath'.)
• An unusually large baby. This may be significant if the second stage is not progressing rapidly in water.

- Situations in which the placenta may not be functioning at its best while there is no sign of foetal distress, there is a possibility that water may be used to facilitate the labour, but birth in the supported standing squat is preferable.

It is common for some faecal matter to be excreted in the second stage as the baby's head descends and compresses the bowel, and the anal sphincter muscles relax prior to birth. If this occurs in the water, the debris should simply be removed immediately with an ordinary plastic strainer. This is a common occurance both in 'land' and water births and there is no evidence to show that this contaminates the water sufficiently to contribute any risk of infection. On the contrary there is a marked absence of infectious complications reported with water births. Some mothers choose to have an enema in early labour to prevent this occurring but it might happen anyway.

POSITIONS FOR UNDERWATER BIRTH

You can give birth underwater in a variety of positions – moving and changing them spontaneously. You could kneel in an all-fours position over the edge with the baby emerging from behind. Alternatively you could squat in the water, holding onto the sides for support. It is much easier to squat unsupported in the water than on land. Your partner could enter the pool as well to support you or he may support you from behind outside the pool by sitting on a low stool or a bean-bag (8). You might choose a semi-sitting position facing forward. Your midwife may decide to enter the pool with you. Some midwives prefer to put on a bathing suit and enter the water, others suggest wearing the cotton trousers and top usually worn in an operating theatre and standing in the pool only if necessary. Most midwives prefer not to enter the pool as it is usually not necessary and quite easy to observe what is happening from the side. The danger of cross infection from the AIDS or hepatitis virus is an issue which arises and has not yet been resolved. Testing in early pregnancy may become necessary to ensure safety. At present rubber gloves are recommended.

BIRTH UNDER WATER

Your baby's head may crown very quickly or it may take some time before the baby is ready to be born. Eventually the head will appear and begin to show through your vagina. You may find that in water it is easier to release your feelings without inhibition and most mothers cry out freely at this stage. The warmth of the water will help to soften the perineal tissues and it is helpful, if you feel like it, to use your own hands to sense what is happening and help the baby to emerge. It is very unusual for a bad tear to occur during a water birth and there is usually no need for the midwife to do anything at all as the baby emerges gently into the water. Often there is no tearing at all. If the body of the baby is not expelled in the contraction following the emergence of the head, gentle assistance can be given by the midwife.

The water in the pool will almost certainly become quite bloody soon after the birth. There is no danger of infection as this blood from the lining of the womb is sterile.

THE THIRD STAGE

Once the baby is born the midwife will check to see if the cord is around the baby's neck and simply unravel or loop it free if it is. If the cord is long enough the baby may well float up to the surface itself or be gently lifted up by you, your partner or the midwife. There is no hurry to lift the baby out of the water and this can be done gently within the next minute or so. Babies have been known to remain immersed for as long as 10–15 minutes after birth but it is generally considered wiser to bring them to the surface within the first two minutes.

Dolphins, porpoises and whales – mammals who give birth in water – usually push their young to the surface to breath within the first few minutes. The baby's breathing response is stimulated by the cooler temperature of the atmosphere on its skin and will not occur until the baby emerges from the water. For this reason, it is important that the room is not overheated for a water birth until after the mother and baby leave the pool. While the baby is still in the water, blood and oxygen will continue to flow through the umbilical cord from

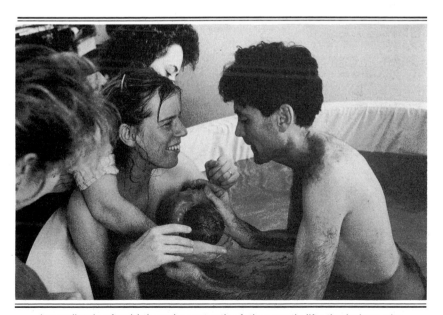

Immediately after birth under water the father gently lifts the baby to the surface and passes him to his mother

the placenta. You or your midwife can feel the cord to reassure yourselves that it is still pulsating and the placenta is still attached.

The baby can then be gently lifted up and cuddled in your arms close to the breast with its face out of the water while the body may remain submerged. The baby rarely has any difficulty establishing breathing because the cooler temperature on the baby's face is enough to trigger the breathing reflex. Very occasionally the baby might need suctioning to clear the nasal passages and this can be done while the baby's body is still in the water. It is not wise to cut the cord as the baby is still benefiting from two sources of oxygen. In the rare circumstance of the baby not breathing it is wise to take the baby gently out of the pool into a cooler atmosphere. This will trigger off the breathing reflex.

First contact with your baby in the water is wonderful as you hold your baby in your arms and look into his or her eyes for the very first time. It is quite safe to remain in the water until your uterus begins to contract again to expel the placenta (usually 10–20 minutes). It is best to be in a vertical position, kneeling or sitting upright so you can hold the baby comfortably at breast level. You will probably find that your baby has a strong rooting reflex and will soon be turning its head to search for the breast. Turn the baby towards you 'belly to belly' to assist the first sucking.

Close attention can be paid to the cord. If it is still pulsating the placenta must still be attached. A decrease in pulse will indicate that the placenta is ready to separate, as well as strong uterine contractions, when the baby sucks. Then it is time to stand up slowly and leave the pool before the placenta is expelled. It is generally considered to be safer to stand up or to leave the pool before the placenta is expelled, to prevent the possibility of water embolism (water entering the bloodstream through any blood vessels that are still open inside the womb). This is a sensible precaution although no incidence of such an occurance has ever been recorded. If the placenta separates unusually quickly before you leave the pool, simply stand up slowly as soon as you realise what has happened. It is not necessary to cut the cord until after delivery of the placenta, but this can be done just before you leave the pool.

Your attendants can help you to leave the pool and have warm towels ready for you and the baby, a warm towelling robe is useful, to put on when you get out. This is the time to increase the temperature in the room and it is important to have an efficient portable heater available so that the room can be made very warm at this point. Once you are outside the pool you can stand up or squat to deliver the placenta and then sit down upright for a while. Make sure that both you and baby are warm and comfortable, while you continue to welcome your baby and enjoy the first breastfeed after birth.

It is possible to bathe the baby in a warm bath after the birth if you wish to continue water immersion or if the baby seems cold, but the warmth of your body is usually quite sufficient. Once the midwife has checked your perineum and had a good look at the baby, you will probably feel like relaxing comfortably in bed with your baby tucked in warmly beside you, close to the familiar warmth of your body.

AFTER THE BIRTH

In the days following the birth much enjoyment can be had by spending time in the pool and this can be a pleasure shared with other family members. Siblings take great pleasure in holding their newborn sister or brother in the warm water and the baby will enjoy the freedom of being in the familiar watery medium while getting to know you and the rest of the family, and exploring the world all around. It is important to ensure that the room temperature is unusually warm, and helpful to keep the lighting subdued for the first day or two. The water in the pool should of course be changed and comfortably warm, but not hot. Newborn babies dislike sudden exposure to the elements so take care to undress the baby slowly in a very warm room and to hold the baby against your body, covered by a warm towel. Enter the pool slowly so the baby makes a gradual transition into the water and the same applies when leaving the pool. It is possible and quite blissful to breastfeed your baby while in the pool, making sure the baby's body is well submerged in the water. The baby can remain in the water for up to 30–45 minutes to begin with, if that feels comfortable, and gradually the time can be extended.

CONSIDERING A WATER BIRTH

When considering the possibility of using water for your birth it is important to keep an open mind and avoid having too many preconceptions or rigid expectations. It is impossible to know ahead of time what will happen. You may find that you do not feel attracted to water at all or that an unexpected complication makes the use of a pool inappropriate. Perhaps the birth will happen so fast that you won't need the pool. On the other hand you may intend to use the pool for your labour only and find that you end up giving birth under water. Some mothers, who planned to use the pool for the birth and then didn't in the end, have derived great pleasure from it in the days following the birth.

Whatever happens, birth is an unknown adventure and it is reassuring to have the possibility of the help of a water pool as and when it is appropriate.

PRACTICALITIES

The water pool to be used for labour and birth should be large enough and deep enough to allow for a variety of positions and the possibility of another person entering the water. It is best when the water is deep enough so that the mother is fully immersed up to just above her breasts when sitting. There are now a variety of water pools available for hire or purchase, and some of these are specifically designed to be portable and can be set up in your own home or in a hospital (9). It is important that the pool is well-equipped with an efficient pump, heater and thermostat. A water thermometer and large plastic strainer to clear the water are important extras. The edge of the pool needs to be padded so that there is a soft wall to lean against and a variety of water cushions are useful.

It is best if the water temperature is approximately 37.5°C or 99°F, i.e. more or less body temperature and comfortably warm. If it is too warm or too cool it may affect labour. Ordinary tap water is quite suitable and no additives are necessary, although some people add salt to the water to create a similar level of salinity as amniotic fluid (1 generous tablespoon per gallon of water). The pool needs to be cleaned beforehand with a mild disinfectant unless disposable liners are provided to contain the water.

PREPARING FOR A WATER BIRTH

The yoga-based exercises recommended in this book are ideal for birth preparation whether on land or in water. It is very beneficial to swim during pregnancy and to spend time relaxing in water everyday, especially in the last three months. Specific water exercises are not essential but you will find that several of the postures you are familiar with can be done under water as well. Gentle breaststroke and swimming and floating on your back are the best strokes to use.

Many women enjoy luxuriating in the bathtub – sometimes more than once a day and the addition of one or two drops of essential oil, such as lavendar, clary sage, tangerine, rose or jasmine, can be very relaxing.

MIDWIFERY FOR WATER BIRTH

Midwives have not yet been trained to use water during labour and birth and may have some queries. Hopefully a hand-held underwater foetal heart monitor will soon be produced, in the meantime the mother may need to stand or sit up on the edge of the pool if monitoring is necessary. Essential internal examinations can be done quite easily underwater with the mother on all fours. The descent of the head can be checked in any position by feeling and the delivery usually needs no assistance but the midwife should be ready if necessary. Unless the second stage progresses well the mother should leave the pool. After the birth hold the baby belly down while passing it to the mother, to help the fluids to drain. When the cord pulsation ceases, it is time to leave the pool. It is important to learn how to bend to avoid backache and a stool is helpful. Contact the Active Birth Centre for details of training or further information.

8 | After the Birth

Your Body after Birth

After the birth, you may be surprised to find that each time your baby sucks at the breast your uterus will contract and, at first, these contractions may be painful. They are known as 'after pains' and feel like strong menstrual cramps. These contractions are helping your uterus to retract back into the pelvis and return to its normal shape and size. After a few days the pains will gradually stop and will be replaced by a feeling of pleasure and well-being as you breastfeed your baby.

You may be fortunate after the birth and find that your perineum is intact with no tear. In this case there may be very little soreness or tenderness and recovery will be quick. On the other hand you may have a graze which requires no stitching or a tear which needs to be repaired. Stitching is usually done soon after you have welcomed your baby and first contact has taken place, and a local anaesthetic is used so that you feel no pain. Generally, a natural tear will heal rapidly in the next day or so and cause little scarring. It is advisable to use the healing and antiseptic herbal bath (see page 196) for a day or two after the birth and this will ensure a good recovery and prevent infection. If you find that there is stinging when you urinate, pour a large jug of warm water between your legs at the same time. Pat dry afterwards with a clean towel and then dab the scar with homoeopathic calendula tincture (neat or 10 drops diluted in a little previously boiled water). Allow to dry before dressing. Do not use ointment or cream as the moistness may dissolve the stitches too rapidly. Use a child's swimming ring to sit on if you are uncomfortable. Later, when the wound is healing (at the itching stage), apply a little vitamin E oil after bathing to prevent scarring and promote healing.

Bleeding from the uterus (known as lochia) will continue for some time – like a long period – gradually lessening until all the blood rich lining of the uterus has been shed. Use soft sanitary towels rather than tampons as these may cause infection.

In the hours after giving birth you will probably find it impossible to fall asleep and need to bask in the 'afterglow' of the birth and go over all the events that have happened, before weariness takes over and you fall asleep. Your baby will probably be very alert for a few hours and then fall into a profound sleep. It is best to keep your baby in close body contact with you for several days and to enjoy an extended 'babymoon', with few visitors for the first week after birth. At least a few quiet days getting to know each other as a family will be invaluable. Your partner will need time and peace to 'bond' with the baby too, as both of you learn how to respond to his or her basic needs. For the next day or two you will probably find that the very special atmosphere that follows the birth continues. It is very easy to 'shatter' this atmosphere with too much disturbance or insensitive intrusion and it is well worth making careful preparation beforehand for these first special days. Many parents who take these precautions report a postnatal 'euphoria' that can continue for a week or two and certainly helps them to acclimatise to early parenthood.

Starting to Breastfeed

Very often, with the prospect of giving birth ahead, we give little thought to breastfeeding. Sometimes, especially after a physiological birth, breastfeeding follows very easily with little or no difficulty. However, more often than not there is a lot to learn and the first week or two can be quite challenging.

It is helpful to understand some basic physiology before you start. In the first day or two after birth your breasts produce a substance known as *colostrum*. This is a thick, yellowish liquid which you may have noticed in the last weeks of pregnancy. This wonderful fluid is the perfect first food for your baby. It is highly nutritious and contains valuable antibodies which fortify your baby's immune system for the future and also help to protect your baby from bacteria in the environment. It also has a laxative quality and clears your baby's digestive tract, preparing it to absorb milk in the days to come. It will help to clear the *meconium* from your baby's bowel. This is a sticky dark green substance that collects in your baby's bowel during pregnancy. After birth your baby begins to defecate for the first time and soon after the birth the first meconium will appear! Gradually, with the help of colostrum, the meconium clears and by the third or fourth day it is replaced by soft yellowish stools. Sometimes the meconium can take a day or two to appear and this is completely normal.

An important reason to keep your baby close to you in the first few days is to encourage the baby to take in as much of the colostrum as needed. Michel Odent, in his book *Primal Health*, stresses the need for the baby to consume 'huge quantities' of colostrum. The baby's sucking will stimulate its production so it is important not to limit sucking time. Additional water or glucose water is rarely necessary for a healthy baby fed in this way, and weight loss is usually negligable. Proper sucking of the colostrum will stimulate the release of the first milk. Just before the milk 'comes in' your baby may be a little fretful and impatient. A few drops of spring water on a clean teaspoon will help to quench his thirst. The milk usually comes in within 2–4 days after the birth and this day is often a little difficult. Your breasts will probably become quite hot and swollen (known as engorgement). This can be very uncomfortable but usually lasts only about 24 hours. You may also find that you are quite weepy and a bit depressed. It may be more difficult for your baby to latch on to the breast during engorgement.

HELPFUL TIPS:

- Lie on your belly in the bath before feeding and massage your breasts gently towards the nipple to express a little milk into the warm water.
- Stand under a warm shower with the water coming down onto your breasts.
- Use warm compresses (face cloth rinsed in hot water).
- If engorgement is very bad, try taking the homoeopathic remedy Belladonna 6x every half an hour until symptoms ease.
- In many traditional societies midwives 'bind' the breasts with a long soft cotton cloth. Using a long scarf instead of a bra may increase comfort, make it firm and supportive but not too tight and wrap around the neck 'halter style' to secure. A 'sports bra' may be comfortable.

How Does Breastfeeding Work?

The first principle of breastfeeding is supply and demand. The amount your baby sucks will determine the supply of milk. Your baby can increase the supply by doing more sucking (which is what is happening on days when sucking seems endless). Milk is produced in little cells which are arranged in clusters within the breast and look a bit like miniature bunches of grapes. When your baby sucks, signals go via nerve endings to your pituitary gland in the brain; a hormone known as oxytocin is released and this makes the milk-producing cells contract and release the milk (it also makes your uterus contract at the same time!). The milk is ejected into little ducts that carry it to the 'ampullae' or reservoirs just behind the areola. You can feel these as little lumps surrounding the base of the areola (the area surrounding your nipple). From there the milk 'lets down' and is ejected via the tiny opening in your nipples. At first there often seems to be far too much milk, but gradually the amount your baby sucks will determine the right supply.

It is important to understand two points:

- The 'let down reflex' may not occur for a minute or two. You may feel it coming on as a tingling sensation in the breast and it may happen as soon as you even think of feeding, but sometimes the signal cycle takes a little time. Therefore it is vital not to take your baby off the breast after a couple of minutes (often mothers are wrongly advised to start breastfeeding for just two minutes on each side). If you remove the baby before the milk lets down, the supply will be discouraged and the milk supply may dry up.
- Positioning your baby correctly at the breast will help to prevent nipple soreness:

a Sit upright in a comfortable chair or in bed. Soon you will also be able to breastfeed lying on your side, with your baby cradled beside you. If you have had a Caesarean you will need to start in this position.

b Make sure you are holding your baby comfortably 'belly to belly' i.e. with baby's mouth facing the nipple and body facing towards yours.

c It is vital that your baby 'latches on' properly. Wait for your baby to open its mouth wide. This may require a bit of tantalizing. When the mouth is wide open, draw the baby towards the breast using your free hand to help offer the breast to the baby if necessary. Make sure that your baby takes in a good part of the areola as well as the nipple. The part underneath the nipple is most important and should be mostly taken into the baby's mouth, unless you have very large areolae. Remember that your baby feeds from the breast and not from the nipple. Your baby will then 'milk' the breast by massaging the ampullae – or reservoirs behind the areola – with rhythmic movements of the lower jaw. Once the baby has drawn the nipple and areola into his or her mouth, the massaging movement of the baby's jaw and tongue stimulates the ejection of the milk. When a baby is latched on properly the nipple will end up right at the back of the throat. To get an idea of how this works try sucking your thumb for a moment. If your baby is latching on properly most breastfeeding problems can be prevented. Some discomfort and nipple soreness can be expected, but continued feeding should 'break in' the nipples and soreness will pass.

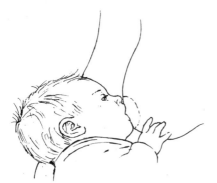

This baby is not latching on properly and is sucking the nipple only

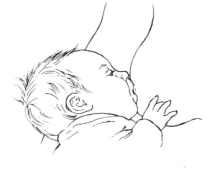

When the baby latches on properly the nipple and part of the areola are taken into the mouth and the lower lip curls under

d Feed your baby according to demand. At first this may seem continuous as your baby has been used to continual feeding in the womb. Gradually a pattern of feeding and digesting will emerge. It is important for your baby to empty the breast at each feed as the milk changes consistency and the most nutritious milk is at the end of the feed.

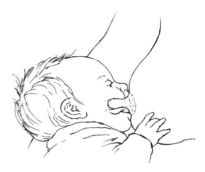

When the baby is correctly attached to the breast the nipple extends to the soft palate. Rhythmic wave-like movements of the tongue draw the milk toward the baby's throat

e Allow your baby to suck until he or she is satisfied. Usually the baby will fall blissfully asleep at the breast at the end of feeding. Babies vary in the amount of time it takes to feed but, as they grow older, feeds are shorter with larger gaps in between. It is best not to time feeds at all.

f If difficulties arise, contact a breastfeeding counsellor from the La Leche League or the N.C.T. as soon as possible (see Useful Addresses). It is wise to make contact with a breastfeeding counsellor near to you before the birth.

Breast Care

The following advice should be helpful:

- In late pregnancy massage your breasts and nipples with almond oil after bathing. Read a good book on breastfeeding (see Recommended Reading).
- Never use soap on your breasts as this removes natural lubricants.
- Don't wash your breasts between feeds. Milk contains natural antiseptics and one bath a day is sufficient to ensure cleanliness. After a feed allow your breasts to dry naturally and then massage a little pure almond oil into the nipples. Expose to the open air for a while before putting on a cotton feeding bra. Choose one that opens in front and make sure it is well fitted by an expert.
- Use washable or disposable breast pads that do not have a plastic backing, and change frequently.
- If soreness occurs use homoeopathic calendula cream after feeds. This will not harm your baby. Expose your breasts to fresh air as much as possible. Mild sunshine for a short period will help.
- If you do remove your baby from the breast, take care to break the suction first by inserting your little finger into the corner of your baby's mouth.

Breastfeeding in the Months to Come

After a week or two breastfeeding your baby should become a pleasure which nourishes both of you. Breastmilk is the perfect food for your baby and will ensure that he or she has exactly the right nutrients throughout the first year. While you may introduce solid food around 4–6 months, if possible, breastmilk should still form the mainstay of your baby's diet until 12 months or longer. There is no food as complete in nutrients as breastmilk. Baby formula made from cow's milk can make an adequate substitute, if necessary, and has been formulated to resemble human breastmilk as closely as possible. However, it cannot entirely imitate the dynamic living properties of breastmilk.

If circumstances allow it is best to bear in mind the following points:

- Feed your baby like a gypsy – without watching the clock and according to your baby's demands. It is not possible to overfeed a breastfed baby. Plumpness is normal in breastfed babies and will be shed when your baby becomes mobile!
- Let your baby lead the feeding. Feeding patterns vary. Your baby may be fed almost continuously in the late afternoons and less in the mornings, or the other way round.
- If possible, let your baby lead the weaning. Breastfeeding can go on for as long as 3 or 4 years and this is completely normal for some mothers and their babies. There are no rules but breastfeeding your baby for the first 6 months is most important. If you can continue for a year, or longer, your baby will only benefit.

9 | Postnatal Exercises

In the first weeks after birth your main concern will be getting to know and taking care of your baby. You will need plenty of rest and a very nutritious diet, and you probably won't have much time or inclination for formal exercising. Many hours will be spent breastfeeding your baby and this is a perfect opportunity to rest, relax and put your deep breathing into practice (see Chapter 3, exercise sequence I, no. 2). However, there are a few essential exercises to do to help your figure to return to normal in the coming months. You will also find a short exercise programme an invaluable way to stay relaxed and to combat tiredness or lack of energy, which are so common in early motherhood.

The essential exercise programme that follows has been designed to be followed in sequence, each exercise gradually strengthening the body in readiness for the next. The exercises begin the first day after birth and gradually build up to a programme for the first six months. Although one week has been allocated for each sequence, it doesn't matter if it takes you 10 days or longer until you are ready to progress. It is important to follow your own rhythm and to fit exercising around the time spent with your baby, which should be your first priority.

The postnatal programme of exercise concentrates on the following areas:
- Toning and firming the pelvic floor muscles and helping the uterus return to normal.
- Strengthening the lower back which carries so much additional weight in pregnancy.
- Toning the abdominal muscles to restore their strength and elasticity.
- Releasing tension in the shoulders and neck – areas which are under stress from the many hours spent carrying your baby.
- Improving circulation to the breasts and maintaining good posture and tone in the muscles that support them.
- Maintaining the increased flexibility and mobility of the joints which you achieved in pregnancy while promoting the tightening of the ligaments.
- Lightening the pelvic area and helping the return to normal curvature of the spine.
- Reducing fatigue and stimulating good energy flow and circulation.

- Relaxation.

Swimming and walking are excellent in combination with the exercise programme and are enjoyable for your baby too! There is no need to diet to regain your figure if you are exercising well and breastfeeding your baby. A sensible nutritious diet which is well-balanced is essential. You will find that many of the exercises are already old friends from the pregnancy programme.

Week 1

1   On the first day or two after birth, try lying on your belly in bed and tightening and releasing your pelvic floor muscles up to 10 times – several times a day. This may become uncomfortable when the milk comes in and your breasts are tender. You can then place a pillow under your ribs or do the exercise lying on your back with knees bent.

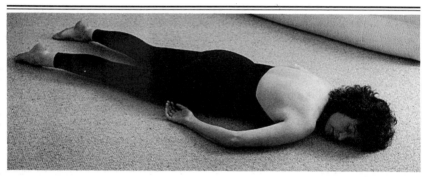

Position for pelvic floor exercise

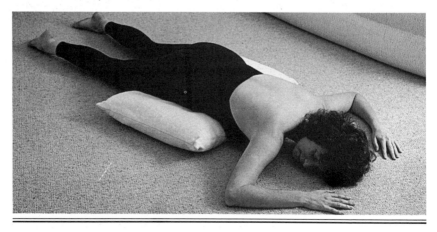

If your breasts are tender, try this

2   Lie on your back on the floor in the basic reclining position (see page 72, exercise sequence VIII, no. 1), with your hands on your belly and knees bent. Breathe deeply as before, but concentrate on tightening the abdominal muscles and drawing them down towards your spine when you exhale, releasing them with the in-breath. Repeat up to 10 times.

3   In the same position, contract, hold and release your pelvic floor muscles 10 times.

4   In the same position do the belly-toning exercise (see page 66, exercise sequence VII, no. 1). It is helpful to start this exercise within a day or so of the birth. Build up to repeating 10 times.

5   In the same position do the pelvic lift (see page 72, exercise sequence VIII, no. 2) and the lower back release to strengthen your spine (see page 74, exercise sequence VIII, no. 3a).

6   Total relaxation – known in yoga as the corpse pose, this is probably the most important postnatal exercise and aids recovery after birth. This should always be done at the end of your exercise session, or on its own. Lie flat on your back with your legs and arms spread comfortably apart. You may place a pillow under your knees if you prefer. Tuck your chin in to release the back of your neck and close your eyes. Breathe deeply in and out through your nose, feeling the movement of the breath in your belly. With each exhalation relax and release each part of your body in turn, remembering to keep your jaw and eyes relaxed. Feel the way the back of your body contacts the floor and let go of every bit of tension with each out-breath, so that your body sinks down with gravity as you relax more and more deeply. Remain in this position for at least 10 minutes, covering yourself with a blanket if you are cold. This should be practised daily for 10–20 minutes and can be as relaxing as a few hours of sleep.

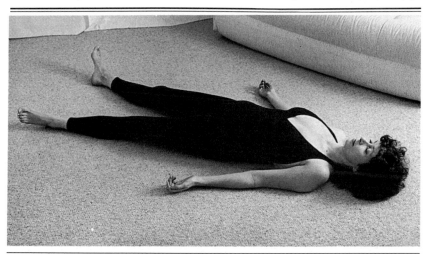

Total relaxation

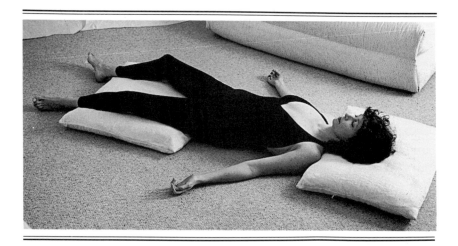

Week 2

Add the tailor pose (see page 39, exercise sequence II, no. 1).
And the pelvic lift (see page 49, exercise sequence III, no. 4).

Week 3

Add kneeling with knees apart (see page 45, exercise sequence III, no. 1).
And the spinal twist (see page 47, exercise sequence III, no. 3).

Week 4

Add the whole of exercise sequence V, the shoulder release (see page 58).

Week 5

Add legs apart on the wall (see page 68, exercise sequence VII, no. 2a, b, c).
And the shoulder stand:
a   Lie on your back with your buttocks close to the wall in the same position as
'legs apart on the wall'. Bend your knees and place your feet together. Relax
your shoulders, place your arms by your sides with the palms down and tuck in
your chin to release and lengthen the back of your neck. Breathe deeply into
your belly and relax and release all of your spine, especially your lower back,
neck and shoulders, onto the floor. *(Caution: When doing this exercise do not turn
your head to the side. If your baby calls, come down and out of the position.)*

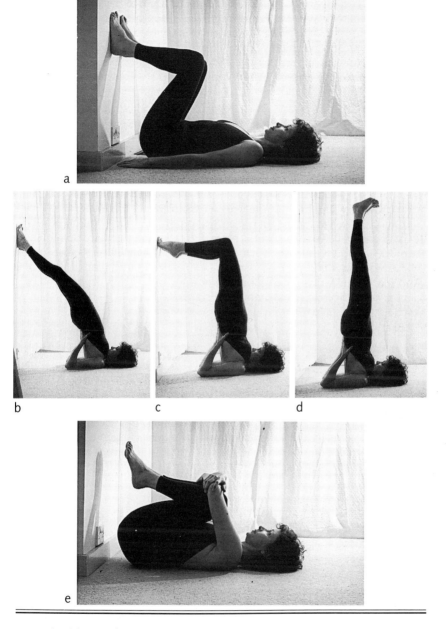

Shoulder stand

b   Tuck your elbows close into your sides and 'breathe' them down onto the floor. Then, keeping them in position, press your feet into the wall and lift your body up, supporting your upper back with your hands behind your ribs. Keep your neck and shoulders relaxed and go only as far as you can without strain. Straighten your legs, keeping your feet on the wall and your elbows down. At first your pelvis will feel very heavy and it will be difficult to place your hands on your upper back, but with regular practice your neck will relax and your pelvis will become lighter. Focus your exhalation on dropping your elbows onto the floor and take it slowly. Hold for a second and then come down slowly on an exhalation. When this becomes easier do 10 pelvic floor toners before coming down, drawing the pelvic floor down towards your navel when you contract, holding for a second and then releasing. Hug your knees (e) before coming up.
c   When (b) becomes easy, bend your knees and press the wall with your feet to bring your pelvis above your shoulders so that your trunk forms a 90° angle with the floor. Make sure your elbows are well tucked in. Place your hands behind your ribs and breathe your elbows down when you exhale. Hold, then relax and release your spine onto the floor gently, and hug your knees (e).
d   This usually takes several weeks but when (c) becomes easy, try straightening your legs to find the balance. Your weight should be supported by your elbows and upper arms while your body forms a 90° angle to the ground. To come down place your feet on the wall and drop your spine gently from the neck.
e   Hug your knees to release your lower back.

BENEFITS

This exercise brings lightness to the pelvic area and aids recovery of the pelvic floor and uterus. After the first few weeks, pelvic floor exercises should always be practised in this position. Practised regularly, this can cure a prolapsed uterus and will reduce varicose veins, haemorrhoids and vulval varicosities. It also releases tension in the upper back, neck and shoulders, and benefits the endocrine system, helping you to regain hormonal balance after birth. You can complete most of the essential exercises in about 10 minutes. If you find you only have time for one exercise sequence start with the legs apart, then the tailor pose on the wall, the abdominal toner and the shoulder stand.

Week 6 – 6 months

As time and inclination allow, add the following to your exercise programme:
Sitting with legs wide apart (see page 42, exercise sequence II, no. 4)
Exercise sequence IV, 'standing positions' (page 51)
Dog pose (see page 61, exercise sequence VI, no. 2)
Exercise sequence no. VIII – spinal release, but omit no. 5 (see page 72)
Always end with total relaxation (see page 157)
In the months to come you will be ready to continue with more advanced yoga. See Recommended Reading and Useful Addresses for contacts.

10 | Active Birth at Home or in Hospital

You will probably be asked to choose the place of birth right at the beginning of your pregnancy, and you may then find that you are expected to stay committed to your original choice (though you are always entitled to change you mind). But it is not always easy to decide at this time as you may not know very much about the whole subject yet, or the options available. Certainly you will not yet know how the pregnancy is to progress, which must influence your choice. Women, like other mammals, have a powerful 'nesting instinct' which usually arises towards the end of the pregnancy. Just as a cat chooses her corner of the house before the kittens are due to arrive, you too may not know where you wish to give birth until closer to the end, though you may have some preferences or ideas.

If at all possible, it is advisable to register for your antenatal care with your midwife, GP or a local hospital and then keep all your options open before you commit yourself and, in the meantime, explore the possibilities. It is possible to change your GP for the duration of your pregnancy or to choose a particular hospital which may not be your nearest, because you like their approach. If you need advice or help concerning your legal rights, then contact AIMS (the Association for Improvement in Maternity Services – see Useful Addresses). It is advisable to pay a visit to any hospital you are considering before committing yourself, to find out about the general approach in the labour ward and whether they encourage Active Birth.

On the other hand, you might prefer to explore the other options available.

Home or Hospital?

There is no way of removing every risk in childbirth. Although the vast majority of babies are born safely, the final outcome of any birth is always uncertain. Unexpected complications can arise, machines can break down, anyone can make a mistake. There is no evidence to prove that either home or hospital is safer. Recent evidence indicates that it is not necessarily safer for birth to take place in hospital – even for a first baby, so it is worth considering carefully which is the right choice for you. Different factors, such as your health, age, whether you have any problems in pregnancy and what choices are available to you, will help to determine the most appropriate place of birth.

The most important thing is to discover all the possibilities, to consider what your priorities are, then to make a choice which feels right for you. Your instinctive feelings are really important and they will arise most strongly at the end of your pregnancy. The choices are:

a A home birth.

b The domino scheme (this means 'domiciliary midwife – in-out'). With this system you are under the care of the community midwives who attend to you antenatally and will come to your house in labour, take you into hospital, and then deliver your baby in hospital and take you home six hours or so later. Postnatally, they will look after you at home. The great advantage is getting to know your midwife beforehand.

   This system can be a good compromise between a home birth and birth in hospital and women enjoy the continuity of care. It is not usually easy to find out whether this service is available but ask your GP, your local hospital or the local supervisor of midwives.

c A GP unit is where you have your baby in hospital but under the care of your own GP with your local community midwives attending you. The hospital would take over only in the event of complications arising and you can go back home after six hours with your baby if all is well. Many women find this a good way to give birth actively in hospital and enjoy the more homely atmosphere and the familiarity of a doctor and midwife whom they know well.

d Then there is the choice of a consultant hospital. (Some of these have some GP beds too.) Nowadays many more hospitals encourage Active Birth and may have a special birthing room available.

If you would like more information and advice on the choices available see Chapter 11 for some useful addresses and contacts. If you have any of the following problems you may need to have your baby in hospital.

TOXAEMIA OR PRE-ECLAMPSIA

This occurs when blood pressure rises to dangerous levels. It does not mean the slight rise in blood pressure which is quite common at the end of pregnancy and which needs careful observation but generally presents no problems, unless it continues to rise or rises sharply. Blood pressure is connected with emotions and sometimes the excitement of approaching the birth can cause a slight rise. (See Chapter 11 for prevention and treatment of high blood pressure.)

BREECH PRESENTATION

There are more risks involved than in a normal presentation. (See Unusual Presentations under Active Birth in Hospital.)

PREVIOUS COMPLICATIONS

Not all complications are likely to recur. However, if there were problems with the last birth which could affect this one then you may be better off in hospital.

PLACENTA PRAEVIA

Sometimes the placenta lies in the lower abdomen and is actually close to or covering the cervix. Here the danger is that the placenta could separate and be born before the baby and result in the baby being cut off from its source of nourishment.

Although a low-lying placenta usually ends in a perfectly normal birth, it may be necessary to have help close at hand in case a Caesarean is required. (With a real placenta praevia, a Caesarean is always necessary.)

Active Birth at Home

'There was a feeling of great calm and peace and relaxation around and we all lay down together in our family bed for the night. It felt so good not to have any separation either from Kurt or David.'

There are many advantages to a home birth. In your own home you are the centre around which everything else revolves, rather than a patient, dependent on the routines of a large institution. Your attendants come into your home as guests. You can relax in the comfort and security of a familiar atmosphere, with your loved ones around you. The birth is an event in your family life, a special occasion, a time to celebrate. For the other children in the family, particularly if they are very young, a home birth is of great value as they can welcome their new brother or sister without having to cope with a separation from you. If all goes well, some families choose to have their children present at the actual birth and, in this way, completely included in the experience.

'As he was born and we were waiting for the cord to stop pulsating I suddenly became more aware of how wonderful it was, for us all to be together at this time – the girls had witnessed the birth of their brother in a very bonding experience.'

In pregnancy you have the great advantage of continuity of care. There is plenty of time to get to know the midwife or midwives, who are going to attend you, and to discuss your wishes with them in advance. You can also have the comfort of your own family doctor being present at the birth. Make the most of the many opportunities to discuss what you intend to do with your doctor or midwife. It will help you to approach the birth with confidence if you feel that you can trust your attendants to support and encourage you to give birth actively. If this is their first experience of Active Birth then lend them this book!

'The prospect of even a small difficulty ahead suddenly daunted me and being at home, in loving arms, made it easier for me to protest that I couldn't face it. In hospital, in being geared to fight off interference, I was also fully geared to fight my own weakness, whereas at home it was safer for me to want to give up.'

If you are hoping for a natural birth, you can avoid routine hospital practices and there is less temptation at home to resort to drugs or intervention in your weaker moments. You are the only person in labour, the birth process can unfold naturally, you can take your time and are not subjected to the inconvenience of moving to hospital. Being moved in labour usually disturbs the rhythm and contractions slow down. You can create the ideal environment, use the bathroom whenever you want to, make as much noise as you want to, listen to music and help yourself to food or drink of your choice. It is possible to have complete bodily freedom and privacy, and to give birth either on your own bed or on the floor. You can be alone or share the experience with people of your own choosing. After the birth, you can all be together to enjoy the special time of celebration in the family. You can sleep when your baby sleeps and have your baby with you in bed, day or night. It is usually easier to establish breastfeeding and to learn to care for your baby in these conditions.

Medically speaking, you are expected to fall into the 'low risk' category, you should be in good health with no problems in your pregnancy and no history of illness or obstetric complications which could affect the birth. Sometimes, however, a mother who is 'high risk' may also be better off staying at home where she is assured of the careful attention of a skilled attendant.

Arrange suitable back-up in advance in case complications arise and you need to be transferred to hospital.

THE BIRTH ROOM

'I went upstairs to the bedroom which I had prepared for the birth. There was a foam mattress in front of the fire, covered with a clean sheet, an enormous bean-bag also covered with a sheet resting against the foot of my bed and a small stool to sit on between contractions.'

Arrange a pleasant environment where you have several alternatives for changing positions. There is no special equipment needed – most homes will have everything you need already. Make sure you have a good supply of cushions and a low stool or pile of books for squatting on.

The room should be warm with extra heating available for the actual birth as the baby will need to be kept very warm immediately afterwards. The lighting should be comfortable. Dim light is most conducive for relaxation in labour, with one lamp or angle-poise light handy for the midwife in case she needs it. Your midwife or local clinic will provide you with a maternity box for the delivery. (Useful for the supply of cotton wool alone.) Having said all this, it is necessary to add that it is quite likely that you will give birth in another place entirely. It is not uncommon for babies to be born on the bathroom floor!

In labour, make full use of the bath tub or shower. It is unlikely that your baby will be born in the water, however it is perfectly all right if it does happen. It is usually best to wait until you are halfway through your labour (about 5cms) before spending long periods in the bath or else you may use up this valuable resource before you really need it (see Chapter 7).

'I decided to relax in a bath. On feeling a contraction I stepped out of it to lean against the sink and to slowly rotate my body as if twisting a hoola-hoop. I continued in this way, topping-up the bath with hot water until I had three consecutive contractions each lasting about a minute.'

A portable sonicaid heart monitor, if your GP has one, will increase the safety factor.

If you decide to have a bath with the baby or to bathe the baby in a baby bath, the water should be warm, as the baby has been used to your body temperature, but not too hot.

After the birth it is not necessary to dress the baby for several days. Have plenty of soft towels or wrapping blankets handy (soft flannel sheets would be fine) as the baby needs to be kept warm. For the first day or two after the birth (or longer), it is best for the baby to be close to the warmth of your body and the familiar sound of your heartbeat. It is perfectly safe for you to sleep together (and to bath together) at this time. This will ensure that the baby gets plenty of the valuable colostrum which contains antibodies to strengthen his or her immunity to bacteria. It also has a laxative effect on the digestive tract and prepares it to absorb the milk which will 'come in' on the second or third day after the birth.

In the hours after the birth your midwife will help to clear up and then she will leave. It's worth thinking in advance of what you will need at that time and have it all handy at your bedside beforehand. Mainly you will need a bowl for warm water and cotton wool to clean the baby when the first bowel movement occurs. This is usually a dark green or black sticky substance called meconium. In a day or so the bowel movement will become a yellowish colour. You will need nappies of some sort. Disposables in the tiniest size are handy and save you having to wash nappies at first. You need plenty of them! It is also a good idea to have some almond oil or calendula cream to put on your nipples after the baby sucks. This will help prevent soreness (see Chapter 8).

You will probably be feeling marvellous after the birth, but take care to be getting enough rest and sleep and to use your energy for your baby. Without the protection of hospital visiting hours, one can find oneself entertaining visitors all day after a home birth. You need plenty of time to get to know your new baby quietly.

If you have difficulty in arranging a home birth then see Chapter 11 for some useful addresses and contacts who may be able to help.

Active Birth in Hospital

There is no reason why Active Birth cannot be put into practice in any environment suitable for birth. Indeed there are many hospitals in London and elsewhere in the country where women who have prepared for Active Birth have managed successfully to give birth in this way. If you are having your baby in hospital, do find out beforehand whether they will allow you to move around and use natural positions for delivery. It is advisable for you and your partner to make an appointment to see the consultant under whom you are booked, and then have your wishes written on your card with his or her consent. Do ask questions about everything you want to know, as many hospitals will be willing to accommodate you. It is wise to talk to the senior nursing officer, who is head of midwifery, as she will be most familiar with the way the labour ward is run. You may want to ask questions such as:

- Is it possible to give birth on the floor rather than on a bed or delivery table?
- Do they have hand-held foetal heart monitors that can be used easily in an upright position without disturbing the flow of labour?
- Do they use syntometrine routinely or do they encourage a physiological third stage? Are they willing to be flexible about this?

More hospitals are recognising the advantages of Active Birth although there are many where the emphasis is on intervention and the use of technology. In some hospitals the staff encourage Active Birth but others may not. It is important for you to find out the situation well in advance and it is your right to change to a hospital which suits your needs. As already mentioned, the domino scheme or GP unit system is often the best way to have an Active Birth in hospital, and has the great advantage of continuity of care and gives you an early opportunity to discuss your wishes with the midwives and your doctor.

'I had previously stated that I wanted no enema, monitor, drugs or cuts unless absolutely necessary and once the midwife had confirmed my wishes, no more was said.'

Whether you are having your baby at home or in hospital you will need good antenatal care and education during your pregnancy.

WHAT TO TAKE WITH YOU

Take a large, firm floor cushion or two (measuring roughly three feet square) or a bean-bag with you to lean on, as the small pillows usually provided by the hospital do not offer enough support. The cushion should be firm, as high as possible and, of course, very clean. You will need several hospital pillows as well. Ask for extra pillows when you arrive.

Most hospital delivery rooms have a stool which is used for getting up onto the bed. This is perfect for squatting. Place one of the pillows on it or ask the midwife for a disposable paper pad. The delivery table is usually quite narrow so it is not ideal but it is wide enough to kneel or squat on reasonably comfortably. The bars at the back of the delivery table come in very handy for holding onto while kneeling or squatting, and if the whole bed is pulled forward by a few inches, your partner can also stand behind the bed to support you.

Most delivery beds are adjustable – they can usually be lowered, the back can be raised and sometimes the end and the backrest can be removed altogether. Explore these possibilities in advance. (We keep hearing from people about new ways in which they have managed to use whatever is available at the time.) If the staff allow it, your partner can sit on the bed with you in order to support or massage you. It is best if you are completely free to move around in labour and have the choice of being on the floor or on the bed. Although the delivery bed is rather high and will restrict your movement to some extent, it does allow you to be easily supported and your attendants can reach and see very easily. Many hospitals are willing to place a mattress on the floor for women who wish to squat or have a squatting birthstool. This is very helpful.

Make a tour of the labour ward beforehand, notice the whereabouts of bathrooms and showers so you can make use of them during your labour. It is also a good idea to take a pad for kneeling on. A piece of foam rubber two inches thick in a clean pillow case is ideal. Then you can kneel on the floor or use it on the bed to protect your knees.

Many couples like to take a tape recorder with music of their choice and this is often quite delightfully relaxing for the attendants as well.

Take your own nightgown to wear as you will want to look and feel good. A short cotton one which can open in front (or a man's shirt or pyjama jacket) is ideal and easy to take off. You will need a sponge (natural if possible) and a face cloth for wiping your face in between contractions, and a fan in hot weather. If the room is overheated (often the case in hospital) try turning down the radiators.

You may like to take your own tea bags for herbal tea (camomile or raspberry leaf) and a jar of pure honey. A spoonful every now and then in herbal tea will ensure that your blood sugar level doesn't drop, and eliminate the need for a glucose drip. Natural apple juice or red grape juice will have the same effect, as will glucose tablets (don't take citrus juice – it's too acidic). Of course, your partner will need some food and some coins for the call box.

MOVEMENTS FOR LABOUR

You will probably be advised to stay at home for the first part of the first stage and hopefully you will arrive in hospital to find yourself already dilating. When you arrive you will be admitted and examined to see how far you have dilated. The position and well-being of the baby will be checked and you may be offered an enema and a bath. It is possible to refuse the enema if you would rather not have one, as it is not necessary. When you arrive in hospital don't be surprised if things slow down for a while – as soon as you relax and settle down, the rhythm of the labour will pick up.

A bath or shower is very relaxing – don't rush, enjoy it! Many labour wards have showers and, if you have a long first stage, you may enjoy making use of them from time to time. You can walk around the delivery room or up and down the corridor. When labour gets stronger you may like to stand at the side of the delivery bed, place your big cushion in front of you and lean forward onto it for contractions, using the stool for one foot. Another good idea is to sit on a chair facing the bed and lean forward onto it.

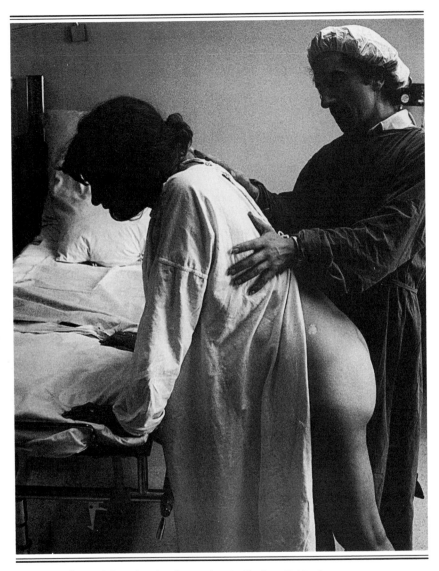

Standing in labour leaning forward on to the hospital bed

You can use the stool for squatting, or squat on the floor holding onto the bar of the bed for support. When labour gets very strong, you can get up on the delivery bed if you are expected or want to do so. Lift up the backrest and pile your cushions up against it so that you can lean forward onto the cushions and rest, completely supported in the kneeling position between contractions.

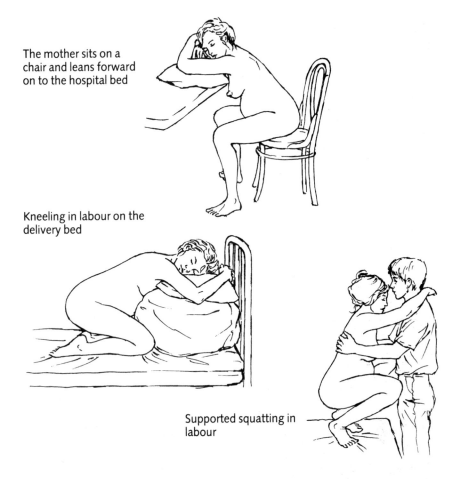

The mother sits on a chair and leans forward on to the hospital bed

Kneeling in labour on the delivery bed

Supported squatting in labour

You can squat holding on to the backrest. Alternatively, your partner can stand behind the bed to support you – or at the side. Try squatting sideways on the bed, putting your arms around your partner's shoulders for support.

You could also face the other way and squat leaning forward. Follow your instincts to adapt the environment to suit your needs.

THE SECOND STAGE IN HOSPITAL

The kneeling position presents no problem on a bed, simply kneel forward onto a pile of cushions. If you are able to remain on the floor you can follow the advice given in Chapter 6 for the second stage. Some hospitals still insist that the second stage take place on a bed. If this is the case for you, these are the ways of being supported in a squatting position on a bed.

Squatting with two people supporting

　　'Very soon after arrival I felt like pushing, was examined and found to be fully dilated. Contractions were now coming almost continuously and I squatted throughout, supported by my husband and an extra doctor who had come along to watch.'

Squat on the bed. Place a pillow under your heels as this will make squatting easier. Your supporters should stand at your sides on either side of the bed. If they are more or less the same height you will probably be able to put one arm round each of their shoulders quite comfortably. They can each put one arm round your back and use the other arm to support you under each knee, if this is comfortable for you. If the second stage takes some time then wait until the baby's head is coming to go into a squat, to avoid becoming too tired.

　　For variation and resting you can come forward into a kneeling position. It is also possible to stand up during contractions by holding on to your supporters' shoulders.

　　'I was helped by the doctor and my husband into a squatting position. This was marvellous! I could push so much easier and it was a comfort to feel their strength helping support me. I stayed squatting as this brought her head down very quickly!'

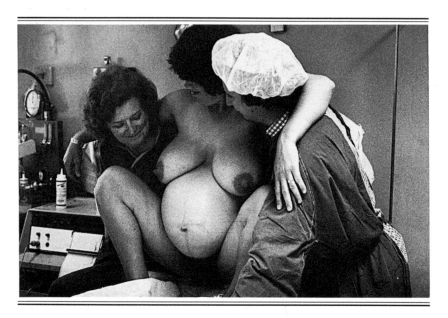

Partners stand at the side of the bed and support the mother in the squatting position

　　Another way to support you in the squatting position is from behind. This works well in a situation where it is possible to lower the backrest. Your partner can stand behind the bed and support you as in the 'standing squat' in Chapter 6.

This can also be done (and is possibly more comfortable) if the mother squats sideways on the bed, if the midwife is willing to assist from the other side.

Birth in the supported squatting position on a hospital delivery bed

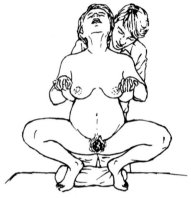

The mother squats between her partner's knees. He sits on a bean-bag behind her on the delivery bed

The partner stands behind the bed while the mother squats

Another possibility is if the supporter sits on the pile of cushions or bean-bag on the bed, behind the mother. Then she can squat between his legs using his body for support. If an upright position is not comfortable or possible, then try a side-lying position in preference to semi-reclining.

These examples are all drawn from situations where people have managed to find their own ways of making use of whatever is available and acceptable to the hospital. It is important to visit the labour room beforehand to get an idea of the possibilities and to discuss them with the staff.

Monitoring the Baby for Active Birth

This means checking your baby's heartbeat and needs to be done regularly during labour. It is possible to hear the baby's heartbeat clearly by placing one's ear against the abdomen. The ordinary ear trumpet is perfectly adequate and the midwife may ask you to sit up vertically or lean back slightly while she uses it. Some enterprising midwives manage to use it from underneath while the woman in labour kneels. The stethoscope is perhaps easier to use in this position. The best type of monitor is the doptone or sonicaid hand-held heart monitor. These are relatively inexpensive and most hospitals and doctors have one. They can be used with the woman in any upright position and cause no discomfort to mother or baby. There is no evidence that the ultra-sound waves used affect the baby but this is still under-researched. There are portable hand-held monitors which can be used at home. You hear the sound of the baby's heartbeat magnified which can be very reassuring.

The abdominal belt monitors most commonly used at the time of writing present certain problems. They involve the mother wearing two belts strapped around her abdomen – one to measure the contractions and one the baby's heartbeat – which generally confine her to the semi-reclining position. Many women complain that these are very uncomfortable. The contractions are more painful and also there is a real contradiction here – the monitors are meant to detect any foetal distress while confining the mother to the position most likely to induce it! Also we know that machines often break down and don't work properly, and when midwives rely solely on machinery their instincts to detect distress suffer. As a compromise to continuous monitoring, some hospitals suggest that you have the belt monitor attached for twenty minutes to obtain a continuous picture. This is usually unnecessary and may be disturbing if you find the belts uncomfortable, although some women do not object.

Women from our classes have successfully used belt monitors in the kneeling position which helps to solve some of the problems.

'I had to get onto the delivery bed and be monitored, as the doctor was worried as the baby was small. As soon as I lay down on the bed the contractions were painful and so as soon as the monitors were attached I turned over and knelt up on the bed. Immediately the pain disappeared and I could cope well with the contractions.'

The other form of monitoring very commonly used, often in addition to the belt monitor, is the scalp electrode. This was designed for use on babies that are at risk and was never intended to be routinely used for normal labour. The electrode is attached by a tiny screw or hook to the baby's scalp through the cervix. This form of monitoring allows the mother greater mobility depending on the length of the flex and the flexibility of the attendants. However, the disadvantage here is that the membranes have to be artificially ruptured in order to attach the monitor, and this has its attendant risks – it will accelerate labour, sometimes violently, and increase the risk of infection. Rupturing the membranes also causes unnecessary pressure from the contracting uterus on the infant's head (see Chapter 11, Artificial Rupture of Membranes). Their effect on the baby, as a first touch from the outside world, is also questionable. Some babies are left with a small wound and occasionally a permanent tiny bald patch where the electrode was attached.

In the event of a real complication, such as the baby being distressed, this form of monitoring may be appropriate as it is considered to be more accurate than a belt monitor and, in such a case, the baby's safety is a priority. If your doctor insists on routine use of this form of monitoring refer him or her to an article in the *Lancet* (page 207, reference no [1]) on scalp electrode monitoring.

There is a new form of radio operated monitor (telemetry) currently being marketed which allows complete mobility but still necessitates rupturing the membranes to attach a scalp electrode.

It is essential that the system of monitoring should not disrupt or disturb the normal physiology of labour. As soon as this is the case the monitor itself can become the cause of the problems it is intended to prevent.

Midwives usually check the foetal heart once every hour or so. When labour is obviously progressing well, the midwife may not need to check the baby's heartbeat as often and may rely on her intuition. In the second stage the foetal heart may be checked more frequently but again this may not be necessary.

Internal Examinations

These are done by the midwife to assess the progress of the labour. She will insert her hand into your vagina and feel the cervix and the top of the baby's head to gather information about the dilation and the presentation of the baby.

When birth is active and labour is obviously progressing well it is not necessary to make these examinations often, and sometimes not at all. Most midwives like to examine internally at the end of the first stage to check if dilation is complete. You may wish to be examined to know how far you have dilated yourself.

Some women do not mind being examined but others often complain that it is uncomfortable to be touched in this most tender part during labour. Internal examinations can be done very gently between, rather than during, contractions and in a position most comfortable to you. It is possible to examine a woman standing up (with one leg up on a chair), sitting on the edge of a chair or kneeling forward on all fours.

'The hospital staff agreed to and managed examinations with me sitting on the edge of a chair. And regularly the baby's heartbeat was checked with a portable monitor – which hardly interrupted me at all.'

This may be far less uncomfortable than turning over into the semi-reclining position.

Usually midwives have been trained to examine in a semi-reclining position and often do not like to change their ways, which is understandable. Perhaps you could ask to try another position first, agreeing to turn over if she has any difficulty and then she will probably discover that it is just as easy. If, for some reason, she requires you to turn around, it cannot harm you to do so and you can turn back again when she has finished. Breathing deeply and relaxing as much as possible while being examined should help.

The kneeling position offers attendants an excellent view of what is happening as the baby is born. In fact, as far as view and access go this position is ideal. The problem here is that the midwife's routine is literally turned upside down – but there should be little difficulty. When dealing with spontaneous birth in which the woman follows her own instincts, the midwife is also, by necessity, more spontaneous and more instinctive. In the few places in the western world where birth is managed this way, the statistics are so much better than those of our high technology hospitals, that there is justification for the argument that spontaneous midwifery is safest and best, and more satisfying for all concerned.

In a squatting position the midwife will need to rely on her hands to feel the baby's progress, or else bend down to look. As the pelvis is more open and perineum more relaxed in this position there is less need for examination and rarely any need to guard the perineum.

After the baby's head emerges the midwife will check with her finger to see if the umbilical cord is round the baby's neck. It is a common occurrence and all the midwife will normally have to do is to loosen the cord by pulling it a little and slip it over the baby's head and body as it emerges, or just after. Midwives with experience of the squatting position tell us that this presents no problems and can be handled in exactly the same way as if the mother was reclining.

In the rare case of the cord being wound twice or more times around the neck, it is safest for the mother to be squatting in this instance (preferably a standing squat), as the pelvis will be wide open and the baby will be born much quicker than if the mother were reclining. She should sit down as soon as the baby is born to help the midwife unravel the cord. Cutting the cord is not desirable in this situation, unless it is preventing the baby from coming out, and in these circumstances a supported standing squat or kneeling position is imperative. Normally, once the child is born, the cord is quickly unravelled and left to stop pulsating while the baby is placed between the mother's legs on its belly in the 'safety' position.

Accelerating Labour

If labour is very slow, there is usually no cause for concern provided the baby's heartbeat is normal, the mother is coping and feeling well, and the labour is progressing. Many women need to take a long time sinking into the first stage, and others need time to let the baby descend to be born in the second stage. In a slow labour, immersion in water after 5cms dilation is often very helpful. Walking (stopping to lean forward during contractions), perhaps outdoors if the weather permits, can help.

Generally, the best way to help a slow labour is to darken the room and leave the mother alone for a while in privacy. Sometimes nipple stimulation can help to intensify contractions.

As far as movement and posture goes, the more vertical postures will help the baby to descend and exert more pressure on the cervix. Squatting is likely to intensify the contractions. Movement will probably accelerate the labour and half-kneeling, half-squatting can speed up dilation of the cervix. It often happens that progress is very slow and suddenly advances rapidly – it could be 12 hours or more going from 0–6cm and 10 minutes from 6cm to full dilation.

Sometimes hunger can cause delay. Perhaps the mother is afraid of something she cannot express, or is struggling inwardly with unconscious inhibitions. If she is given understanding and space she will probably find her own way of overcoming her difficulties.

It is quite normal for some labours to stop and start during the first stage. If labour is not progressing after a long time has elapsed and there does not seem to be an obvious reason, one should allow for the possibility that there may be some physical problem, such as the presentation of the baby or the internal shape of the mother's pelvis, and help may be needed.

Slowing Down Labour

If labour is progressing very fast then the kneeling position on hands and knees can help the woman to stay in control. The knee-chest position may help to slow down the contractions (see page 110). Very slow deep breathing can be helpful.

Unusual Presentations

Usually before the birth, the baby lies with its head engaged in the pelvis in what is known as the anterior position. The baby's back will be lying against your abdominal wall and the limbs will be folded in front facing your spine. The head will be flexed well forward ready for birth. In this position the baby's descent through the birth canal will be easiest. However, sometimes there are variations in the way the baby lies.

With the use of natural upright positions these variations can usually be managed without intervention. When the mother is moving in labour there is more likelihood of the baby being able to move into the correct position.

POSTERIOR PRESENTATION

This position is fairly common and may be caused by the position of the placenta. Babies like to face their placentas *in utero*, so if the placenta is on the front wall of the uterus, the baby may be lying posterior.

In the posterior position, the baby is lying with its spine against your spine and its limbs facing towards your abdominal wall. Usually the baby will rotate into the anterior position just before or during labour, but sometimes remains posterior for the birth. With the use of upright positions this doesn't usually present any serious problems, however there is more pressure from the baby's head on the mother's sacrum, which usually results in a 'backache labour'. The fit between the baby's head and the pelvis isn't quite as perfect so the labour can be somewhat slower. The instinctive way to deal with a posterior presentation is to kneel forward so that the weight of the baby is taken off the mother's back, which eases the pain. In this position, the heaviest part of the baby, i.e. the spine and back of the head, will tend to gravitate downwards and this will encourage rotation into the anterior position. Rotating the hips will help the baby to descend. Standing up, leaning forward and rotating the hips is also useful.

For the second stage, squatting or a standing squat are best, allowing maximum opening of the pelvis and help from gravity. Sometimes the kneeling position is most comfortable and practical for the delivery.

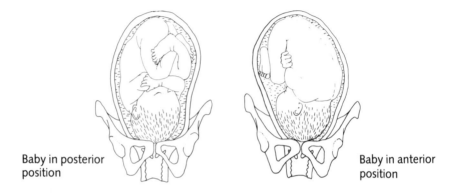

Baby in posterior position

Baby in anterior position

BREECH PRESENTATION

When a baby is lying in a breech position, its head is uppermost and its bottom or legs are presenting first.

It is quite possible for a baby to be born in this position but there are ways of gently encouraging a breech baby to turn before labour starts. It is desirable to do so as a breech birth may be problematic in that the head of the baby is the largest part of its body and will be emerging last. If there is any delay this can be dangerous.

With an Active Birth the risks are minimised and, provided the first stage goes well and a supported standing squat is used, most breech births are uncomplicated. However, it may be difficult to find an obstetrician who has experienced vaginal breech birth in an upright position, and interventions such as forceps and a Caesarean section are sometimes recommended routinely when a baby is breech. Most babies lying breech will turn of their own accord before the birth. This may happen just before labour starts. Walking for an hour a day in the open air will encourage the baby to turn. The head is the heaviest part of the baby's body and will move down towards gravity – encouraged by the walking motion.

If you discover that your baby is breech by 35 weeks, stop squatting and try this exercise having discussed it first with your doctor or midwife. A word of caution – lots of babies are lying breech 6 weeks before birth and then turn spontaneously, so don't do anything until 5 weeks beforehand (i.e. 35 weeks).

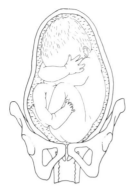

Breech presentation

Exercises to encourage a breech baby to turn
(Caution: If you find that you are dizzy lying on your back then you should not do these exercises – try to spend time in the knee-chest position instead, see page 110.)
It is important not to use force but to attempt certain movements oneself, which may gently persuade your baby to turn. If the baby insists on remaining in the breech position then allow nature to take its course. First of all discuss this exercise with your doctor or midwife and ask them to help you to feel how your baby is lying before you start. Discover the exact location of the head, the limbs, the baby's spine and the placenta, if you can.

TRY THIS:

Place a large firm cushion or two on the floor and lie down on your back with your hips raised up on the cushion and your head on the floor, so that your pelvis is higher than your head. You can place a pillow under your head if you feel breathless.

Exercise to encourage a breech baby to turn

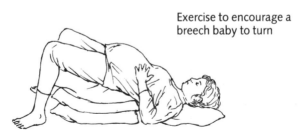

In this position the baby will drop slightly away from the pelvis and may begin to move. Lie like this for ten minutes several times throughout the day. Relax and breathe deeply. Massage your belly with your hands and try, gently, to encourage your baby to turn. Ask your midwife or doctor which would be the easiest way for the baby to turn and massage in that direction only, so your hands give the message to your baby. Use a vegetable oil on naked skin so you can massage easily. Use gentle but firm and consistent pressure. In many ways this is a matter of communication between you and your baby, and it usually takes a week or two before the baby turns. When it happens you will probably feel that there is a change. Arrange beforehand with your doctor or midwife that as soon as you suspect that the baby has turned you can have an examination. If this confirms that the head is down, then stop doing the exercise and start squatting in order to help the head to engage.

Homoeopathy and acupuncture can assist a breech baby to turn. One single dose of homoeopathic remedy pulsatilla (10m) will stimulate the baby to move, as will a simple acupuncture treatment called 'Moksha', applied to a point on the little toe. With Moksha, heat rather than needles is used and this can be done by an acupuncturist while you are lying in the position above. If your partner accompanies you to the session, the acupuncturist can teach you to continue the treatment at home. Use homoeopathy and acupuncture in combination with the exercise and daily walks.

Usually after this a baby will turn. However, if your baby is still breech in labour, then, if your obstetrician is agreeable, stay vertical and squat fully to bear down in order to give your baby as much room as possible and to get maximum help from gravity.

Michel Odent stresses that in the case of a breech the supported standing squat is imperative for delivery as it allows for rapid descent of the baby through the pelvis. Odent believes that this method of delivering a breech is safer than a forceps delivery where there is always a risk of damage to the baby from the forceps. Very rarely, in order to speed up delivery of the head, an episiotomy can be done (while you remain standing) just before the baby's head emerges (see Episiotomy, page 181). If the first stage does not progress satisfactorily, the baby will need to be born by Caesarean section. However, it is generally not necessary to do a Caesarean until there has been a trial of labour. If the baby needs help in second stage, forceps are usually used.

TRANSVERSE PRESENTATION

If your baby is lying transverse by the fourth week before labour is due, then do the same exercise as for breech. Kneeling and rotating your hips for the first stage may help to get your baby into the correct position. If the baby remains transverse, a Caesarean section will be necessary but it may well turn head down at the very last minute. It's worth a try! Walking for an hour every day may help the baby's head to descend.

There are a few very rare instances where the baby's head is at an unusual angle, with the neck extended rather than flexed. This can lead to a situation where the head cannot pass through your pelvis. However, this is less likely to happen if you are moving your own body intuitively during labour.

It is most important to have a thorough pelvic examination in early pregnancy as it is helpful to know that the shape and size of your pelvis does not present any difficulty. This is supposed to be part of the routine check in early pregnancy but it is often overlooked in the busier antenatal clinics.

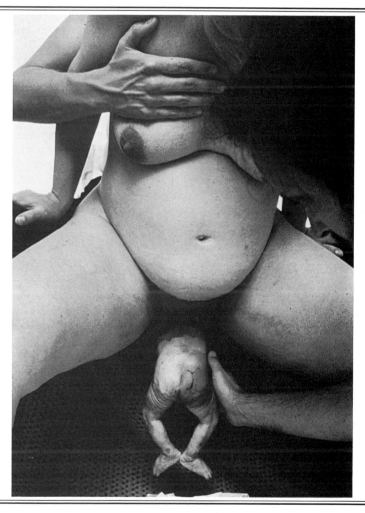

Breech presentation
Upright supported squatting is essential to maximise the help of gravity when a baby is born actively in the breech position

Perineal Tears

In the second stage of labour, as the baby's head comes down to the base of the pelvis and crowns, the perineal tissues between the vagina and anus fan out and stretch open. In the squatting or kneeling position, the pelvis opens to its widest and the back or sacral part of the pelvic floor draws backwards and is in a passive state of relaxation, allowing maximum opening of the vagina. In this position a tear is less likely than if you are reclining. However, tears are a natural hazard of birth. They usually heal without difficulty and the stitching to repair them can be done with a local anaesthetic.

HOW TO AVOID A TEAR

- During pregnancy practise yoga-based exercises and pelvic floor exercises regularly.
- In the last six weeks you could massage the perineum and the whole vaginal area with olive oil after your bath. Some midwives recommend stretching the perineum with your fingers. These are traditional practices in many cultures but your perineum will soften naturally anyway.
- Use upright squatting or kneeling positions for the birth of the baby.
- Don't rush or push forcefully in the second stage. Let your uterus be your guide and follow your own urges to deliver your child. If you don't try to hurry the process your perineum will generally have time to fan out and relax.
- Ask the midwife not to swab you down with disinfectant as this simply washes away the natural lubrication and will make a tear more likely.
- In natural positions it is generally not necessary for the midwife to guard the perineum. However, if the tissues seem very tight it is very helpful to apply hot compresses. A small towel (a good way to break in the new nappies) or a face cloth can be used. Take several and pour almost boiling water over them in a basin. As soon as they are touchable, wring one out and fold it, having let it cool down (test it on your wrist), place it on the perineum. Use a new one after each contraction. This is very soothing and will help to bring blood to the area and relax the tissues. In hospital a quick compress can easily be made by using a sanitary towel and hot water from the tap. Squeeze out excess water and apply. Your partner or midwife will need to prepare the compress. They should feel warm without burning.
- Use your own hands to feel the baby's head when it begins to crown and to ease the tissues or even massage them with a little oil. Interestingly, mothers who use their own hands to help the baby out rarely tear!
- Feel free to shout spontaneously as the baby emerges – as your throat releases, so will your perineum!
- Giving birth in a darkened room with as few people as possible, so you can let go without feeling 'watched', is the best way to avoid a tear.

REPAIRING A TEAR

Sometimes a small tear will not need stitching. If it does, however, it is definitely advisable to have a local anaesthetic to deaden the pain as this is not going to affect your baby. Make sure you don't feel anything and ask for more anaesthetic if you do – even one stitch can be very painful without an injection. Also, ensure that whoever is doing the stitching has plenty of experience and can do a good job. (See Chapter 11 for a marvellous herbal remedy to soothe and promote healing in the days to come.)

It is not necessary to have your legs up in stirrups while a tear is being repaired and, in fact, you can probably relax better with your legs apart and knees bent.

Episiotomy

An episiotomy is a surgical incision or cut which is made in the perineum with scissors to enlarge the vaginal opening. A local anaesthetic is injected into the area beforehand so that the incision is painless. You will not feel the incision being made, but you will probably have some discomfort afterwards while it is healing. The cut is roughly ½–1 inch long and is made through the skin and muscle of the perineum, either down the midline or at an angle, and is sewn up after the birth (whereas a natural tear is more superficial and does not go through the muscle layer).

The need to intervene in this way is certainly the exception rather than the rule but, with the advance of modern obstetrics, episiotomy has become a routine procedure and it is now done in this country to the majority of all first-time mothers, and between 30–70 per cent of all deliveries.

In 1981, the National Childbirth Trust published a booklet on episiotomy edited by Sheila Kitzinger, which is essential reading for any mother-to-be and her attendants (see Chapter 11, Useful Addresses). The results of their survey show that generally episiotomy is unnecessary and that a natural tear heals better and presents fewer physical and psychological problems than a cut. In our work we have exactly the same findings.

When birth is active and natural, upright positions are used for the second stage, and when the mother is encouraged to take her time and follow her own instincts, rather than to push forcefully, the need for an episiotomy is greatly reduced. It is only in rare situations, where the perineum is especially tight, or if an episiotomy will be life-saving for the baby by speeding up the delivery, that it is really necessary. When birth is active episiotomy takes its rightful place as an emergency procedure.

In combination with Active Birth, the 'all fours' kneeling position is the best posture to use when an episiotomy is required. In this way the baby is receiving a better supply of oxygen as there is no pressure on the internal blood vessels, the mother is more comfortable, the perineal tissues are most accessible and relaxed and there is less danger of extended tearing after the cut is made, as there is less pressure on the perineum when the baby's head emerges. If the baby is distressed the greater opening of the pelvic outlet in this position would help to speed up the delivery. It is important, if you have an episiotomy, that the stitching be done soon after the birth to prevent blood loss, infection and to promote healing. Local anaesthetic is essential.

Many professionals now recognise that episiotomies are performed unnecessarily. However, the routine use of this intervention is still widespread. It is the most common of all obstetric operations and is often done without the consent of a healthy woman, who may not need it at all. As the after-effects can be very painful and the actual operation, though brief, can disturb and interrupt one of the intimate and deeply personal experiences of your life, it is well worth discussing this subject with your attendants before the event and having your wishes written on your medical card.

> We obstetricians teach that episiotomy prevents tears and reduces the likelihood of prolapse in the future – but we have little or no evidence for making these statements. Not only is there no evidence that episiotomy prevents tears but there is some evidence to the contrary. . .
>
> M. J. House, MRCOG, Consultant Obstetrician,
> from *Episiotomy – Physical and Emotional Aspects,*
> National Childbirth Trust, 1981.

Active Birth and Obstetrics

It often happens that women manage successfully to combine Active Birth with obstetric help. Here are some examples.

INDUCTION

With Active Birth the need to induce labour artificially is reduced. However, if you have symptoms of pre-eclampsia or if your baby must be born without delay – that is, if induction is medically indicated – then prostoglandin suppositories or oral syntocinon are best for active labour as they will not restrict your movement. Normally, once labour is induced, careful monitoring is necessary. If vaginal suppositories do not work, a drip can be applied in the kneeling position and this will be very helpful to you in coping with the contractions, which are often far more intense and violent than the natural ones. Some hospitals have mobile drips which enable you to walk or stand up. The heart monitor can also be worn in this position (see also Chapter 11, Inducing Labour).

'Although my son's birth was induced, I found plenty of opportunity to use the all-fours position, using a rocking motion during contractions and resting back on my heels with knees well apart, and meditating in between.'

You will need to have a good pile of cushions or a bean-bag to support your body in the kneeling position so you can rest in between contractions.

EPIDURALS

Side lying is preferable to semi-reclining, but change sides from time to time. You can sit upright and lean forward slightly or sit on the edge of the bed and lean forward with the midwife's assistance. Changing positions is extremely beneficial as epidurals often cause loss of muscle power and therefore less efficient contractions. The reclining position may also reduce bloodflow to the uterus so changing sides will help to prevent foetal distress. For delivery, side lying is preferable to lying back or, if the epidural has worn off, you may be able to manage supported squatting or kneeling.

There have been several cases of women who have decided to use epidural anaesthesia after a long or difficult labour and have then given birth squatting and enjoyed a spontaneous second stage. However, you need to be helped into the squatting position by your attendants. In one recent case where the baby's heartbeat was dipping, it returned to normal as soon as the mother was upright and she gave birth completely naturally. In this case the midwife said that squatting saved the baby from a forceps delivery. If you want to give birth squatting, it is best that you have a low dose epidural (which can always be topped up if necessary) so that it wears off at the end of the first stage. When you are fully dilated, your attendants will need to get you off the bed and onto the floor to support you in an upright squat. This will greatly increase your chances of a spontaneous vaginal birth and make it easier to bear down.

The use of a water pool for strong labour is the best way to avoid needing an epidural (see Chapter 7).

FORCEPS OR VENTOUSE

These are instruments used in the event of an emergency to help your baby out.

Forceps are like metal salad spoons with a hole in the middle that the obstetrician can insert on either side of the baby's head to help it out, and a ventouse or vacuum extractor attatches by suction to the baby's scalp to help ease the baby from your body.

Often the use of pain-relieving techniques such as epidurals weaken the power of the uterus so that forceps or ventouse are needed to extract the baby. While ventouse is favoured in most European countries, forceps are more popular in the UK. However, sometimes there is a choice, though it is difficult to assess which method is less disturbing for the baby. Ventouse is certainly better for the mother as pain relief and episiotomy are not needed, as they are with forceps.

If you have an Active Birth you are less likely to need pain killers. By using standing, squatting or kneeling positions the need for forceps or ventouse is greatly reduced. Often, after an Active Birth, the midwife has commented that if the woman had been lying down she may well have needed the help of forceps. Occasionally an unusual presentation, a sudden rise in blood pressure or the baby being distressed would necessitate the use of forceps or ventouse. Although this has never been tried, at the time of writing, it seems that the 'all fours' position would be far better for these procedures than the usual reclining position, for the following reasons:

1 No compression on blood vessels, so there is more oxygen to the baby.
2 Greater opening of the pelvic outlet and more help from gravity.
3 Maximum relaxation of the perineum.
4 More efficient contractions.
5 Greater comfort to the mother.
6 Easier access.

Active Birth and Medication

Any drug you take in labour or pregnancy will filter through the placenta and enter your baby's bloodstream. None of them will do your baby any good. Opponents of natural childbirth say that they are not prepared to 'allow' nature to take its course unimpeded until it is proved to be safer than high technology. Despite this, almost all the drugs used in obstetrics have never been subjected to properly controlled, scientific evaluation and found to be safe regarding their effects on the development of the child (both at birth and in the long term). The research that has been done clearly indicates that when drugs are used routinely for normal childbirth, rather than as backup treatment, they can sometimes have damaging effects on the mother and child and on the bonding between them after birth (see Chapter 1).

WHEN BIRTH IS ACTIVE

- there is less need for analgesia
- discomfort and pain are less
- the uterus functions better so artificial stimulants are not usually necessary
- labours are shorter
- the supply of oxygen to the baby is improved
- there is less need for forceps or ventouse
- the secretion of hormones which regulates the whole process is not disrupted

Despite the readily available research on these findings the majority of women in this country are still confined to bed in labour, administered drugs and hooked up to a foetal monitor. Birth is still artificially induced and stimulated as soon as there is the slightest deviation from the average. This 'active management of labour' is usually done with the best of intentions to mother and child, in the name of safety.

Undoubtedly there are always situations where medication helps to improve the experience and the safety factor. However, it is certainly worth asking whether it does more harm than good when used routinely. Given that the majority of births are uncomplicated, there is certainly not enough evidence in favour of the use of drugs to justify an overall policy.

Confining a woman to bed in labour increases her need for pain-relieving drugs and artificial stimulants. Almost every woman given the freedom to move in labour has reported afterwards that when she lay down she was astonished how much more painful the contractions were.

'The only times the pain was extreme were those when I lay on my back for a pelvic examination by the midwife. I don't think I could have managed without any drugs if I had been lying down, as when I had to in the early stages it was unbearable.'

There are very few women who could go through labour on their backs without pain relief. Preventing a woman in labour from using her own instincts to find comfortable positions causes the need for pain killers and other drugs. The use of natural upright positions and immersion in water during labour throws a new perspective on the whole issue.

SOME POINTS FOR REFLECTION

It is important to be able to make an informed choice when contemplating the use of drugs. The application of drugs is very well described in the literature on childbirth (see Chapter 11, Recommended Reading) but often some of the well-known disadvantages are not mentioned.

Valium
Causes amnesia (loss of memory) in 70 per cent of all women who use it and passes rapidly to the baby.

Pethidine (see Chapter 1)
Depresses the breathing response of the baby. A baby that has had a lot of pethidine may have difficulty establishing breathing and could suffer oxygen deficiency (particularly if the umbilical cord is cut immediately). An anti-depressant may be given to the baby to counteract the effects of the pethidine. The baby may need to be resuscitated (given oxygen and helped to breathe). Pethidine also has the following reactions:

- It can disturb the baby's sucking reflex, resulting in a sleepy baby, and cause problems establishing breastfeeding which can last for several weeks or result in failure.
- The pain relief is not very efficient unless given in large doses and then it often makes the mother drowsy, nauseous and less able to cope (particularly if it is mixed with a nausea suppressant which is usually the case).
- It works quite well as a muscle relaxant and can help dilation if given in small doses (25–50mg).
- If given too late in labour (after 7cm), the effect can be to ruin the second stage and will affect the baby more by remaining in its system for several days after the birth, when it does not have the help of your body to clear away the toxins.
- If mother and baby are drowsy first contact and bonding are disturbed.

Bupivacaine

- Used for epidurals and gives efficient pain relief from the waist down in most cases, without loss of consciousness. This is especially helpful for Caesareans where it would not need to be administered for a prolonged period and will have less effect on the baby. In this case it facilitates a good bonding as the mother is not unconscious.
- An epidural reduces the muscle tone of the uterus and bladder so that they function less efficiently. A catheter is usually inserted into the urethra to help empty the bladder. The reduced efficiency of the uterus increases the need for delivery by forceps by 20 per cent (using active upright postures for the second stage after tailing off the epidural at the end of the first stage would help to lower this percentage).
- The mother misses the pleasurable feelings as well as the pain, and may not be able to push her baby out spontaneously.
- Epidurals don't always work properly, sometimes they 'take' only down one side and are sometimes not easy to insert.
- There are after-effects such as headaches which can last for a week after the birth.
- Very rarely a wrongly administered epidural can result in paralysis.
- Blood pressure is lowered which can result in less oxygen to the baby and long periods in the reclining position, necessary for an epidural, also diminish the oxygen supply. If blood pressure falls too low the mother may become faint and dizzy.
- The lowering of blood pressure can be useful in cases where it is dangerously high.
- Research shows that although the condition of the baby after an epidural is much better than with pethidine, epidural anaesthesia can cause either a nervous, jittery or a floppy, drowsy baby.
- The effects of this anaesthetic on the baby are still unknown but it enters the baby's bloodstream and brain cells within minutes. Some recent research indicates that it could interfere with the development of the baby's brain and nervous system, which is taking place during the period surrounding labour and birth (see references for Chapter 1).

Gas and Oxygen (Entenox)

- Enters the baby's system and the effects are still under researched.
- Taken in large amounts it can make the mother feel nightmarish or detached and 'out of her body'.
- A few whiffs in transition help some mothers cope with the worst contractions. However, often the gas and air causes a feeling of confusion and may delay the expulsive reflex.

Trilene

- Has a cumulative effect and can make mother and baby very drugged and sleepy.

Paracervical block
- Affects the baby immediately and makes its heartbeat slower which can result in death of the baby in extreme cases. For this reason it is not used very often in Britain.

Syntocin or Oxytocin drip (see Chapter 1)
- Is used to stimulate uterine contractions and artificially induce or accelerate labour. The contractions are usually more powerful and closer together than in normal labour. If the contractions are very strong they can interrupt the normal blood flow to the placenta and this is more likely to result in foetal distress.
- There is a greater likelihood of the baby being born premature and needing special care, so that bonding will be disturbed. A premature baby is more at risk and is more likely to develop severe jaundice.
- The contractions are more violent, often they have two peaks and are more difficult to cope with.
- A failed induction can result in a Caesarean section.

Syntometrine
- An intramuscular injection routinely used to induce the third stage. This necessitates immediate clamping of the cord and controlled cord traction, increasing the risk of a placental fragment remaining, which may cause infection.
- It interrupts final blood exchange through the placenta before breathing is fully established so oxygen supply is reduced.
- Strong contractions followed by clamping may overtransfuse the baby.
- Risk of neonatal jaundice is increased and the normal processes of the third stage are reversed.
- May make mother feel nauseous and, very rarely, worse complications such as inversion of the uterus can occur.
- Best given intravenously after birth only in those rare cases where a lot of bleeding indicates possible haemorrhage.

When there is a complication or life is at stake, obstetric intervention and medication provide a safety net. Often this can be combined with Active Birth to the advantage of mother and baby. Used routinely, medication can cause problems and can have harmful effects both physically and psychologically.

Stillbirth

In the case of a stillbirth, active labour has many advantages. It assists the mother to have a spontaneous birth, without the use of drugs, which sometimes proves to be very valuable as the mother feels she has gained something from the experience and may be able to use all her knowledge again in a future birth. She may not have a live baby, but she has had a labour. This can be a positive side of the experience. Also, if she delivers in the kneeling position, it gives her and her attendants time to prepare for her to see and hold the baby, which she may want to do. She will recover faster and feel physically well which will help her to cope with the emotional pain that is inevitable after such an experience.

Additionally, if the father of the baby is with her, the experience will probably enhance their relationship which can only help.

'Looking back over my two pregnancies, my overwhelming impression is one of peaceful well-being. In both cases I started exercising regularly at about three months and experienced a growing satisfaction as I reached towards my body's potential. My first pregnancy sadly ended in a stillbirth, but, on being encouraged to use all the positive elements gained from the classes, I tried for and achieved as good and natural a birth as possible. I feel sure that this helped enormously towards my ability to accept and live with the pain of the loss. How glad I was on giving birth to my second baby that I had had this first good experience.'

A Note to Birth Attendants

'My consultant's innate confidence in the normal workings of a healthy body was a real factor for calm and confidence both during my pregnancy and at the birth.'
If you are presented with this book by a woman who would like to put its teaching into practice, I hope you will enjoy helping her to do so. It is hoped that the practice of Active Birth will help to make the atmosphere within the hospital more homely for those families who prefer, or for medical reasons choose, to have their babies in hospital. It is possible to combine some of the psychological advantages of home with the security of hospital by making a few basic changes. What is needed mainly is the right attitude towards the woman.

'There was a lovely Malaysian midwife and a girl student (whom I had already met). Both were friendly and said "Do whatever you like." Ditto the sister in charge of the labour ward, whom I knew from the time of Michael's birth, since she had been on the postnatal ward – she remembered and welcomed us, and offered to put a blanket on the floor if I wanted to carry on using my cushion.'
It is essential that the mother in labour should not be considered as a patient. The attendants should regard themselves as her guests, there to assist her in giving birth, which to her is a very special occasion in her sexual, social and emotional life. While carefully observing the progress of mother and baby, the attendants should try not to disturb the natural process of the birth. Interference should be kept to an acceptable minimum to ensure safety. This means that both mother and midwife will rely more upon their instincts and intuition. Research has shown that whether at home or in hospital, when birth is regarded as natural and instinctive and interference is minimal, safety statistics are impressively better (i.e. in Holland and Pithiviers, France). With Active Birth the art of midwifery comes back into its own and midwives can become more spontaneous and flexible in their approach.

'I was taken straight into the labour ward and was given a big cushion so as to save

my own from being soiled. Only one midwife was present and she let me do what I wanted, helping me squat, advising me on breathing and massaging me.'

THE BIRTH ROOM

Here are some helpful ideas:
- Curtains which can be drawn to darken the room
- Dimmers on the lights
- A bean-bag or pile of large cushions with attractive colourful covers
- A comfortable stool for squatting – perhaps a wooden birthstool
- A comfortable armchair
- A casette tape recorder or record player (or suggest more people should bring their own)
- Sonicaid heart monitor
- A hot water-bottle
- A kettle
- A washable non-slip yoga-mat makes an ideal surface for the mother to stand or squat on for the delivery (see Useful Addresses)

Water is so helpful to mothers in labour that the birth room in hospital should include a bathroom and shower, or at least free access to those that already exist. Ideally a small pool, or double size bath (rather deeper than usual) would be extremely helpful. (For portable water pools which are available for hire or purchase, or permanent pools which can be installed for use in hospital, contact the Active Birth Centre, see Useful Addresses.)

If a bed is used in a birth room it should not be too high or narrow. A low platform with a firm mattress is most comfortable. It should be remembered that furniture in a delivery room dictates how one should behave. If the first thing a woman sees on entering the room is a delivery bed, she immediately feels she ought to get onto it, and is already a 'patient'.

It will help the mother greatly to feel at home if she is encouraged to use her body freely during labour and delivery, and is free to give birth on the floor if she chooses to. A clean sheet with the usual sterile paper pad can be placed between her legs when the birth is imminent, alternatively, a firm mattress could be placed on the floor or a non-slip yoga mat.

In strong labour and transition, the mother needs privacy in order to surrender and open up, and distractions should be minimised, especially as the second stage is starting. Routine examination to check dilation is usually unnecessary. In the second stage women rarely need to be given instructions but should be encouraged to let go, pushing when they feel like it. It is not necessary to use the delivery position until the head is actually crowning (see page 116).

In labour, necessary checks on the dilation and foetal heart can be done, with the minimum of discomfort and interruption to the mother, in a position in which she is comfortable. It is important to bear in mind that a dilating cervix is also the most tender and vulnerable part of a woman's body and the seat of her deepest feelings. It is of great comfort to some women, and their husbands, if they can bring a close woman friend or relative to the birth if they choose to do so. The emotional support is doubled and this also helps the staff. If the woman has other children it is advisable to have them in very soon after the birth (within the first hour) to facilitate bonding.

Immediately after the birth it is helpful and encourages a good bonding situation if the essential checking of the infant is done while in its mother's arms. Then the family should be left alone together with the discreet presence of the midwife nearby for at least half an hour and brought a cup of tea. The baby should be left naked but warmly wrapped up in a soft flannelette sheet so that the mother is free to explore her child. More detailed examination of the baby and stitching of tears can be done after this, if all is well.

Separation after a momentous occasion like a birth can be traumatic for a couple. If it were practical and possible for the father to stay for the first night or first few days this would help many families to enjoy their first hours together as a family, and would have great psychological advantages.

'When everyone had gone and I lay bathed and clean between clean sheets with my man asleep on one side of me and little baby in my arms, I felt a supreme sense of peace and rightness with the world and the laws of nature.'

Working in a busy hospital where birth is a daily occurence it should be remembered that for the family concerned it happens only once or perhaps a few times in a lifetime. The woman rightly needs to feel that she is the centre of what is happening, that this is her day. Her privacy and the profound and intimate nature of what she is experiencing should be respected at all times.

Midwifery is, to a large extent, a social profession – one is working with a family in childbirth or with a couple who are becoming a family. To the woman in labour, the midwife is extremely important. If she feels her to be a friend, someone she can totally trust and relax with, the labour will progress better and will be a better experience for all concerned.

'Sue, our midwife, arrived very quickly, also a close friend. Their warmth and gentleness made us feel calm and very confident.'

Many of the factors to be considered are of a psychological and social nature. Naturally the primary concern to the midwife is the safe delivery of a healthy baby to a healthy mother. By encouraging mothers to give birth actively, you will be helping them to achieve this in a way which is both safe and satisfying.

Should you wish to contact other professionals who have experience of attending women giving birth actively, see Chapter 11 for some useful contacts and addresses.

The exercises recommended in this book for mothers would also help attendants to be comfortable in kneeling and crouching positions in which they can assist a woman squatting (see also Recommended Reading, Chapter 11).

It is helpful to wear trousers for an Active Birth. Some midwives find the white 'theatre suits' ideal for this purpose. Take care to protect your back while bending or squatting – bend your knees or use a very low stool. The physiotherapist at your local hospital may be able to help you find suitable stress free positions.

11 | A–Z Reference

ALCOHOL

Taken in excess alcohol can harm your baby. The occasional glass of wine is all right. In labour alcohol will stop contractions – it is used to prevent threatened miscarriage.

ANAEMIA

If you are anaemic your baby may suffer because less oxygen is carried to the placenta. You are also more likely to bleed heavily after birth and are more prone to infection.

Eat plenty of protein foods (liver is especially high in iron), leafy green vegetables, dried apricots and take vitamins B, B12 and C. A tonic such as Floradix, which contains absorbable iron (or else iron tablets prescribed by your doctor), would help. Floradix is available from health food stores. It can also be helpful to consult a herbalist and/or homoeopath, as there are remedies which can help anaemia.

ARTIFICIAL RUPTURE OF MEMBRANES (ARM/AMNIOTOMY)

This is done by inserting an instrument like a crochet hook through the cervix and breaking the membranes which surround the baby. The result will be that the amniotic fluids drain away and the contractions usually intensify. This is sometimes done to induce or accelerate labour and in some hospitals is a routine procedure on admission.

Normally the membranes break spontaneously before, during or at the moment of birth. Most commonly they break towards the end of the first stage. There is usually no need to rupture artificially – in fact there are some disadvantages in doing so:

- The wedge of fluid between the baby's head and the contracting uterus is lost so there is more pressure on the head and on the cord from the powerful contractions of the uterus. This can cause a decrease in the flow of blood to and from the baby and there is some evidence which indicates that the baby's heart-rate slows down slightly.
- There is also increased risk of infection as the intact membranes and the amniotic fluid provide protection.
- The contractions can suddenly be much stronger and more painful after an ARM, and it can be very difficult to cope with this rapid increase in intensity.
- The baby is probably more comfortable with water between its body and the powerful contractions of the uterus.

However, sometimes amniotomy is carried out because there are signs of foetal distress (such as irregularity of the heart-beat), and it will help to assess the condition of the baby by checking the colour of the water. If the water contains meconium (the first bowel movement of the baby) it is stained green or brown. This can be an indication that the baby is distressed. It is possible to observe the amniotic fluid without puncturing the membranes using an instrument called an amnioscope. In order to attach a scalp electrode heart monitor it is necessary to rupture the membranes first.

Early rupture of membranes

If your membranes break before labour starts there is increased risk of infection as you do not have the protective barrier of the sealed water bag around the baby. Usually infection does not occur and contractions will start up after a few hours, but sometimes it can take longer. If contractions have not started after 12 hours the risk of infection is greater, but many women go for several days before labour starts without getting an infection.

To prevent infection you must keep very clean, washing down after each visit to the toilet. Don't lie in the bath – rather take a shower or kneel upright in the bath to wash down. (It's all right to lie in the water if you do have contractions.)

Garlic tablets and vitamin C will have a naturally antibiotic effect and prevent infection without harming you or your baby. Take 7–8 garlic capsules and 1 gm vitamin C every 2–3 hours till you go into labour.

Treatment with acupuncture can be a very effective way to start labour. Make sure the acupuncturist is experienced in working with pregnancy and birth. If labour does not start within 24 hours, your midwife may be able to help by massaging the cervix to stimulate the release of prostoglandins or by giving you a dose of castor oil and an enema. It is best to avoid internal examinations as they increase the risk of infection.

Signs of infection are a vaginal discharge with an unpleasant smell or a fever.

BACKACHE

Contrary to popular myth backache should not be an inevitable part of pregnancy. As pregnancy advances, your joints will soften due to the release of hormones and your body will need to adapt to the increase in weight. If backache arises it is because there is an underlying structural imbalance which you may not have been aware of before you became pregnant.

The exercises in this book will help to alleviate or prevent backache, but if it persists, it is essential to consult an osteopath who is experienced in working with pregnant women. Pain can be experienced in the lower back, in the sacro-illiac or hip joint, or in the middle or upper back. Other pains that are common occur in the pubic joint, inner thighs close to the groin, rib cage, head and neck, sinuses and also in the wrists. All of these can be helped by the recommended exercises and also by consulting a good osteopath (see Useful Addresses).

BLEEDING

Sometimes in the first three months slight bleeding or spotting can occur at the time you would normally have had your period. This is usually no problem. However, as bleeding of any sort in pregnancy could indicate a possible problem, you should rest in bed, stop exercising and inform your doctor immediately. A small amount of spotting or bleeding is usually no cause for concern. If you have a serious problem with bleeding it is probably better not to do any exercises at all, to be on the safe side. There are homoeopathic and herbal remedies which may be helpful.

BLOOD PRESSURE

Blood pressure is the term which refers to the pressure exerted by the blood on the walls of the blood vessels. The systolic pressure is measured when the heart is contracted and is pushing the blood out and the diastolic pressure is the pressure in the arteries when the heart is relaxed between beats. It is written systolic/diastolic, like this for instance: 115/70. Normal systolic pressure ranges from 100–125 with some variation and the diastolic is usually between 60 and 80.

Eating a good diet, with enough protein, and exercising during pregnancy will help to maintain normal blood pressure. Your blood pressure will be checked throughout pregnancy and labour. A slight rise is fairly common at the end of pregnancy but if the diastolic figure in the reading rises by as much as 15 you are considered to have hypertension. This need not necessarily, but can be, a symptom of pre-eclampsia or toxaemia which is a possible complication of pregnancy.

The symptoms of pre-eclampsia, in its mild form, are high blood pressure with oedema (swelling) and protein in the urine. If you have toxaemia then it may be safest to have your baby in hospital. Sometimes, with bed-rest and good diet, mild pre-eclampsia will improve. The latest research reveals that it is not wise to cut out salt but more helpful to eat extra protein. The problem here is that you feel perfectly well but all the same the condition does need attention.

Very rarely these days does pre-eclampsia lead to eclampsia. The symptoms are headaches, dizziness, irritability, nausea, visual disturbances and pain in the upper abdomen.

If there is protein in the urine it can be a sign of failure of the placenta and may result in premature labour or deprivation to the baby, which is why medical experts prefer to induce labour when there is persistent pre-eclampsia.

Sometimes hypertension is related to emotional stress but not necessarily. There are homoeopathic and herbal remedies which help high blood pressure.

If you are confined to bed it will help to get up every few hours and do some relaxed yoga-based exercises for half an hour and then return to bed. This will help you to exercise your body, and keep up your morale, while possibly lowering your blood pressure.

BREASTS
To prepare your breasts during pregnancy simply massage them with a little almond oil (or any other vegetable oil) after your bath. Don't use soap on your nipples as this tends to dry up all the natural oils. Wear a comfortable, well-fitting supportive bra which is preferably made of cotton. The National Childbirth Trust (see Useful Addresses) stock bras which are ideal for maternity wear. In the days after the birth when your breasts fill up with milk, you will find one of these very helpful.

BREASTFEEDING
It is important to learn about breastfeeding and babycare before you actually go into labour. An Active Birth, followed by good bonding in the first hour after birth, is the foundation of a good breastfeeding relationship. When the natural physiology is undisturbed then one event will flow into another quite naturally (see Chapter 8). However, there can be problems with establishing breastfeeding in the early days and sometimes one needs good advice quickly. Contact the La Leche League or your local NCT breastfeeding counsellor while you are still pregnant (see Useful Addresses).

Recommended reading:
The Motherly Art of Breastfeeding, La Leche League (new English Edition); *The Experience of Breastfeeding* by Sheila Kitzinger; *Touching* by Ashley Montague.

BREECH POSITION
See Chapter 7, Unusual Presentations.

CONSTIPATION
The best remedy is squatting, lots of it. Also eat bran and dried fruit, such as prunes for breakfast. There are herbal and homoeopathic remedies too. Make sure you are taking enough fluids and that your diet contains plenty of vegetables, raw fruit and salads. All starches should be whole grain as refined starches tend to be very constipating. Make sure you follow the urge to defecate when it happens as delay could cause constipation. Walking and exercising daily are important.

CRAMP
This occurs in the legs and no one knows for sure what causes it, but lots of exercise (see exercise sequence VI, no. 1, page 60) usually helps to eradicate it. When seized by a cramp, extend your heel, bringing your toes up towards your body and rub the muscles vigorously. Sometimes when you begin stretching cramps in the foot are common in the kneeling position. Eventually, with practice, this will pass. Calcium supplements may be helpful (make sure these are combined with magnesium and are lead free).

DRUGS
See Chapter 10, Active Birth and Medication; also Chapter 1.

DUE DATE
As some women have longer or shorter menstrual cycles, some have longer or shorter pregnancies. Your due date is only the estimated average – two or even three weeks either way is not uncommon. Late for dates alone (without any other sign of complications) is not a good reason for inducing

labour. It is a good reason for careful observation and for testing the placental function (see Placental Insufficiency). However, this is usually not necessary until 14 days after the estimated due date. Similarly, if you go into labour two or three weeks before your date, your baby will not necessarily be premature (see ARM, page 191).

EATING IN LABOUR

When you are in labour your body tends to want to empty itself of its contents. It is not a good idea to eat large meals or indigestible foods. On the other hand if you have a long labour you are going to need some food to sustain you or you may become exhausted. When this happens, you feel very low and wasted and labour can cease to progress well. Medically it is known as being 'ketotic'. If your urine is tested and contains acetone then this is a sign of ketosis.

Most hospitals do not allow a woman in labour to eat anything at all (in case you need a Caesarian), but prefer to attach you to a glucose drip to avoid ketosis. The disadvantage is that this usually means that you are immobile and restricted to the reclining position, and also you may be hungry! Ketosis can be avoided by the following:

- In early labour eat a light meal, such as a slice of toast, an egg, yoghurt with wheatgerm and honey, or some soup.
- If you are hungry during a long labour eat another light breakfasty snack, or a few spoonfuls of light nourishing soup might be enjoyable.
- Have some form of sugar every now and then, such as a spoonful of honey in boiling water or herb tea, or some red grape or apple juice. If you do become slightly ketotic take some glucose tablets and drink sips of fruit juice (not citrus fruits) between every contraction. Once you are in strong labour sips of water are all you will need or want.
- Make sure your husband or partner has some food to take into hospital as he is unlikely to be offered any in a busy labour ward.

EMERGENCY BIRTH

If you are alone with a woman who is about to give birth and are unable to reach a midwife or doctor then:
- Try to relax and stay calm. Take a few deep breaths with good long out-breaths. *Surprise births are usually completely straightforward.* All you need to do is concentrate really well on what is happening.
- Comfort the mother and, if there is time, reassure her by holding her for a minute or two. Suggest that she go on all fours on her hands and knees or into the knee-chest position, while you get everything ready. Give her a large cushion if there is one. This will help to slow down the contractions a little and will help her to feel more in control and will calm her.
- Get some clean towels, sheets and a duvet if possible to cover the mother and baby, also a towel to wrap the baby in.
- Close all windows and try to warm the room as mother and baby need to be kept very warm.
- If there is time, boil a kettle and switch it off while you wash your hands really well. Get a glass of water, a bowl and toilet roll or cotton wool.
- Go back to the mother, massage her lower back gently and calmly. Give her sips of water and plenty of reassurance. Place a clean sheet, or towel or newspaper underneath her and have some more handy. Have something nearby to wrap the baby in. Place it near a heater to warm up.
- Once you can give her your undivided attention she can stay in that position or else squat against a cushion or bean-bag. Any position she chooses will be all right. If there is no time to think about it any spontaneous position will do, otherwise use all fours.
- All you have to do is concentrate and watch carefully for the appearance of the baby – your instincts will do the rest.
- Allow nature to take its course. Encourage her to take her time and open up, and give way to what is happening inside her. If she panics breathe deeply with her, concentrating on the OUT-BREATH. Suggest that she breathe the baby out rather than push forcefully. Remind her to relax and *slow down.*
- If she is nauseous or sick, don't worry. This is quite normal and is just part of the expulsive reflex.

- If any faeces come out of the mother's anus wipe it clean with toilet paper – away from the vagina.
- As the baby's head emerges support it very gently in one hand.
- The baby may come out in one contraction or else over several. Receive the baby without pulling. Allow her uterus to do all the work, and just let the baby emerge into your hands. Allow the head to hang down a little as this will help the shoulders to come out.
- If the cord is around the baby's neck this is quite common and perfectly normal, simply place the baby down gently on its belly on a soft towel on the floor or bed. Then calmly free the cord from the baby's neck or unravel it as soon as you can.
- If the mother is squatting, hold the baby face down between her feet for a half a minute or so to drain the fluids and then let the mother pick him up in her arms.
- If she is on all fours then receive the baby. Hold it face down for a moment and then pass through her legs to the mother.
- The mother should sit upright with her baby. If a lot of fluid has come out of her then she could possibly move over to a clean sheet or towel.
- Keep them both warm with duvet, towel, coats, whatever you have to hand. The baby's head should be covered too.
- Sit down and enjoy a few peaceful moments with mother and baby. Encourage the mother to place her baby to the breast as this will stimulate the uterus to contract. Don't leave the mother alone in the house.
- Telephone for a midwife or doctor to come round.
- If the placenta comes out between the mother's legs place it in a bowl. Don't cut the cord as it will stop pulsating and clamp itself spontaneously.
- After the placenta is out the uterus should contract down and feel like a grapefruit. If it doesn't then you or the mother should massage her belly firmly to stimulate the uterus to contract.
- If you have some, give the mother some arnica or rescue remedy and perhaps a cup of tea with sugar or honey.
- Use the previously boiled and cooled water from the kettle to wash the mother's genital area, although it is best if she can squat over a bowl of warm water and do it herself. Then give her a sanitary towel or clean towel to place between her legs and a pair of clean knickers.

If the birth takes place in a taxi or some unusual place, then your priorities are to stay relaxed, reassure the mother, catch the baby and keep them both warm.

FLUID RETENTION (OEDEMA)
This is seen as a slight swelling or puffiness in the ankles and fingers and is fairly common in late pregnancy. Homoeopathy can be very helpful in reducing oedema. It is usually nothing to worry about if your blood pressure and urine are all right, but you should report the matter to your doctor. As soon as the birth is over the oedema disappears. Don't cut out salt or fluids, but do eat well – plenty of protein, fresh fruit and vegetables, and whole grains. If the puffiness is severe it may be a sign of pre-eclampsia (see Blood Pressure).

Exercise sequence II, no. 4, will help to reduce the swelling. You could do it several times a day and keep your feet up when relaxing (see Chapter 3).

FOETAL DISTRESS
This happens when a baby is not getting enough oxygen and is usually indicated by the following two symptoms:

1. A baby is distressed when its heart rate falls or rises and is consistently lower or faster than the normal limits of 120–160 beats per minute.
2. When a baby lacks oxygen in labour its anal sphincter tends to relax and some of the first bowel movement (meconium) passes into the amniotic fluid, turning it brown or green. Meconium staining is not always a sign of distress but, coupled with irregularity of the heartbeat, it is very likely that the baby is in trouble. If the baby inhales meconium into its lungs it can congest the lungs and cause respiratory problems.

It is not necessary to rupture the membranes to check if the amniotic fluid is meconium-stained.

Some causes of foetal distress
- Compression of the major internal blood vessels (as in the reclining position)
- Prolonged labour
- Premature induction
- Large doses of analgesic such as pethidine which depress the mother's nervous system, diminishing the flow of blood to and from the baby
- Placental misfunction
- Prolapse, entanglement or compression of the cord
- Diabetes or toxaemia of the mother

Ways to avoid or alleviate foetal distress
a   Keep active and upright during labour
b   If the heartbeat of the baby is irregular try changing positions to vertical or kneeling
c   If foetal distress occurs in the second stage then upright standing squat is the best way to get the baby born quickly
d   It may be necessary to use forceps, ventouse, episiotomy or Caesarean section to help a distressed baby

HAEMORRHOIDS (PILES)

These are like varicose veins which occur in the anus. Do 50 anal tightening exercises (like pelvic floor exercises only concentrate on the anal muscles) in the morning before you get out of bed, and 50 at night before you go to sleep. Use the 'knee chest' position when doing your pelvic floor exercises. Consult a homoeopath and make sure you aren't constipated. For extreme or protruding haemorrhoids don't do full squatting – use a stool instead. Try homoeopathic ointments or compresses of calendula or witch hazel. Ask your doctor's advice too.

HEADACHES

These can occur more frequently in pregnancy. Eat well, get plenty of sleep and don't overdo things. If you feel a headache coming on do the head and neck exercises (see exercise sequence IV, no. 2, page 52). Do some stretches to loosen your shoulders (see Chapter 3). Breathe deeply and relax in a darkened room for a while. You should inform your doctor if you have severe or frequent headaches. Osteopathy can be very helpful.

HEARTBURN

This is very common in pregnancy and is usually caused by a softening of the valve between your oesophagus and your stomach by hormones (the same hormones that soften your joints), so that your food tends to rise up. Eat several small meals rather than one large one and avoid acidic foods. Try some stretches (see page 58). Make some umeboshi juice: take 3 umeboshi plums (from a health food store), boil in a pint of water and keep the juice in the fridge. Drink a little when you have heartburn. The homoeopathic remedy Nux Vom 30 can be helpful when heartburn is severe but don't take it routinely. Avoid eating for three hours before going to bed at night.

HERBS
Herbal teas
Especially good for pregnancy. You can mix them together to make a taste you enjoy or have them separately.

Raspberry leaf (good for uterus)	Fennel (aid to digestion)
Camomile (soothing)	Lemon verbena (delicious)
Rosehip (vitamin C)	Lime Blossom (soothing)
Nettle (excellent iron rich tonic for the blood)	

Herbal bath for after birth
A soothing, healing antiseptic miracle for perineal tears, grazes or episiotomies.

Ingredients: Shepherds Purse
              Uva Ursi
              Comfrey
              6 whole heads of garlic   (Enough for 2 lots)

Method: Take three heads of garlic. Do not peel but prick all over with a fork. Put in a large saucepan with a generous handful of each of the herbs. Fill up with water and bring to the boil. Simmer gently for ½ to ¾ hour. Squeeze the juice out of the garlic with a fork or masher and then cool it. Strain the liquid into a large jar. Put half of the liquid into a shallow warm bath and sit in it for a while. Use once or twice daily. (Use Calendula tincture as well and put some in water to wash yourself after you urinate.)

Herbs available from good herb and health food stores.

HOMEBIRTH
Finding out about home birth
First ask your GP if he/she does home births. If not then ask for referral to a GP who will. If there isn't one contact the Area Nursing Officer (at the city or county health department) to get a list of GPs who do home confinements. Also tell the Community Nursing Officer that you want a home birth and ask her advice.

If that fails write to your Community Health Council Area Nursing Officer and Family Practitioner Committee (addresses from the health department). By law a midwife, called when you are in labour at home, must attend. Also try ARMS, AIMS and SSHC (see Useful Addresses).

HOMOEOPATHY
Homoeopaths recommend certain remedies for pregnancy and labour. The following are generally recommended but consult a homoeopath for any special problems.

The Pregnancy Programme, devised by John Damonte, a famous homoeopath, is suitable for general use by any woman who is pregnant and wishes to ensure that she and her baby will be fit and strong throughout pregnancy, delivery and breastfeeding. These are tissue salts which promote the body's own metabolism. It is not necessary to take iron tablets if you take this programme unless you are anaemic.

Once daily take one of each:
2nd and 6th month: CALC FLUOR 6x + MAG PHOS 6x + FERR PHOS 6x
3rd and 7th month: CALC FLUOR 6x + MAG PHOS 6x + NAT MUR 6x
4th and 8th month: CALC FLUOR 6x + NAT MUR 6x + SILICA 6x
5th and 9th month: CALC FLUOR 6x + FERR PHOS 6x + SILICA 6x

Amongst other things, CALC FLUOR promotes elasticity of vessels and tissues, diminishing the risk of ruptures and lessening the chances for episiotomy; MAG PHOS helps to deal with heartburn and digestive problems; FERR PHOS stimulates the process of absorption of iron preventing anaemia; NAT MUR helps to keep a proper balance in the fluid distribution, while SILICA strengthens both the mother's and the baby's bones and sinews.

Homoeopathy can help with many of the minor complaints and discomforts of pregnancy such as nausea, water retention, heartburn, high blood pressure etc., as well as existing chronic conditions, but it is necessary to consult a practitioner before taking remedies (see Useful Addresses).

There are a few remedies which are helpful to all women in labour, which anyone can safely take without consulting a homoeopath. They do not clash with other medication or drugs, and are of benefit to the baby as well.

Arnica 30x
This remedy is very helpful for pain relief. It also reduces bruising, shock, fear and bleeding. It will help to soften internal tissues and prevent swelling. Take one every half hour or so as soon as contractions begin to be painful or as needed. Continue taking after the birth 3 times daily if you are feeling sore or bruised.

Aconite 30x
This is the remedy to take if you are fearful or anxious. Take half hourly in labour or as needed.

Kali Phos 30x
Towards the end of labour if you feel tired or exhausted this remedy will help. Take half hourly or as needed.

Bach Rescue Remedy

A composition of five flower essences, rescue remedy is very effective when pain or panic becomes overwhelming during labour. Take 10 drops in a little water or a dropperful directly into your mouth. This remedy is particularly helpful in transition. A dropperful can be placed in your drinking water throughout labour. If your partner feels queasy this is a good remedy for him too.

Calendula Mother Tincture

This remedy is a healing antiseptic – use instead of synthetic antiseptics. Put 10 drops in an egg cup of warm water, that has been boiled, to clean baby's cord. Put 10 drops in a bowl of warm, previously boiled water to bathe stitches (do this after you urinate in the days after the birth). Apply neat, using a warm sterilised natural sponge, to stitches in the days after birth. Calendula cream (not ointment) is soothing for sore nipples.

Use throughout childhood to treat infection, cuts, grazes and wounds. There is also calendula talcum powder – useful for the cord and for drying baby's creases.

Belladona 6x

This remedy is useful on the first day that the milk 'comes in' to ease engorged breasts. Take one half hourly when symptoms are severe.

Common teething problems may be relieved by chamomilla (in the potency prescribed by your homoeopath). Other common problems such as colic and rashes may be helped homoeopathically. There are soothing and healing homoeopathic ointments such as Hypercal or Calendula and a wonderful ointment for burns which should be in every medicine chest. A kit of all the above is available by mail order from the Active Birth Centre (see Useful Addresses).

INDUCING LABOUR

See Chapter 7. Labour usually happens when the time is right. More natural ways of inducing labour are: (a) Love-making, there is natural prostoglandin in the semen which softens the cervix, and the relaxation and orgasm may help to start you off. (b) Exercise. (c) An enema. (d) Castor oil (must be prescribed by your doctor). This will cause diarrhoea which may stimulate the labour. (e) Go out and enjoy yourself – have a glass or two (not more) of wine. (f) An acupuncture treatment. (g) Gentle massage of the cervix by your midwife to stimulate the production of natural prostoglandins by the tiny glands in the cervix. If the membranes have ruptured it is best to avoid internal examinations as they increase the risk of infection.

INSOMNIA

Is there anything worrying you which is keeping you awake? Have a warm bath and do your exercising before going to bed. Drink camomile tea in the evenings. Consult a homoeopath. Calcium supplements are sometimes helpful. Insomnia is common in late pregnancy. A warm bath and milky drink may help you to fall asleep – or else get up and do something and sleep later when you feel tired.

INTERNAL EXAMINATIONS See Chapter 10.

IRON See Anaemia.

JAUNDICE

About half of all babies get mild jaundice in the first week of life. They look a little suntanned. It is caused by the baby's liver still being a little immature and unable to cope completely with the breakdown of bilirubin. Premature babies are more prone to jaundice. The baby should be put to the breast a lot as it needs the fluid. Sunlight will be helpful. Some experts believe that not clamping the cord until after delivery of the placenta can reduce the incidence of jaundice. Studies show that there is no advantage in giving the baby water or water and glucose. Unrestricted breastfeeding and sunlight are the best remedies. In extreme cases phototherapy is needed.

KETOSIS See Eating in Labour.

MISCARRIAGE

If you have sudden bleeding, pain in the abdomen or contractions, go to bed, phone your doctor immediately and have a drink of brandy or whisky. Many women miscarry at some time. However, it will take some time to get over a miscarriage and grieving is normal. It is advisable to practise yoga before your next conception and seek emotional counselling if you feel you need it.

MONITORING See Chapter 10.

MORNING SICKNESS (NAUSEA)

Start exercising every day and consult a homoeopath. Homoeopathic remedies such as petrol or sepia can be very helpful but you need the right one for your constitution. Eat small meals frequently and have some milk and a cracker as soon as you wake up in the morning. Morning sickness usually passes by the end of the first three months. Tea with a slice of fresh ginger may be helpful. Morning sickness may very well occur at other times of day. Slippery elm tea is helpful for some women or a drop of essential oil of peppermint on a sugar cube may help.

OEDEMA See Fluid retention.

ORGASM

In pregnancy love-making and orgasm are as beneficial to you as ever. Some women do not want to make love when they are pregnant and some do more than ever. Gentle love-making can't harm your baby. Try different positions, i.e. kneeling on all fours, the knee-chest position, lying side by side like spoons, penetration from behind, etc., to avoid any weight on your belly. Towards the end of pregnancy you may find more shallow penetration or masturbation more comfortable. Nipples become more sensitive in pregnancy and love-making is the very best way to prepare for breastfeeding.

This is a great time to experiment and try some new ideas!

PAIN See Backache.

PILES See Haemorrhoids.

PLACENTAL INSUFFICIENCY

To avoid this eat well during your pregnancy. If this is suspected then ask for tests to be done.

The oestriol test examines the amount of oestrogen in your blood and urine. If the oestrogen is high then it's possible that your placenta isn't functioning well. If you have no other symptoms other than being past your due date placental insufficiency is unlikely.

If your baby is small for dates, zinc supplements are helpful but should be taken at a different time of day to iron.

POSTERIOR PRESENTATION See Chapter 10, Unusual presentations.

RHESUS FACTOR

The Rh factor is found in the red blood cells.

Most people are Rh positive (Rh+), 15 per cent are Rh negative (Rh−). If you are Rh− and your man is Rh+ chances are you are carrying a RH+ baby. If your baby is Rh+ and his blood mingles with yours (which doesn't usually happen) then you would develop antibodies. You will have blood tests during pregnancy to see if you have any antibodies. If your blood is clear and this is your first baby then there is nothing to be concerned about. Your baby's blood is most likely to mingle with yours at birth (it only happens rarely anyway) and by the time you have developed the antibodies the baby will probably be born. So it wouldn't affect a first baby.

A sample of blood from the cord can be taken at birth and if the baby is Rhesus+ then within 72 hours of the birth you should have a Rhogam injection that will prevent you developing antibodies which, if untreated, could affect your next baby. This substance is an extremely useful obstetric drug. Before this was invented the Rhesus negative woman could have had great difficulties and sometimes her baby would have needed a complete blood change after birth to clear the antibodies.

Provided you have no antibodies in your blood, the pregnancy and birth can take place without any cause for concern. If there are antibodies you would need to deliver in a hospital.

SEX IN PREGNANCY See Orgasm.

SPORT

Continue with any sport you already play provided you feel all right about it.

Squash should be avoided as the hard ball could damage your baby. Walking, dancing, jogging (in moderation, and only if you are used to it) and cycling are all suitable, particularly walking, and swimming. The latter is especially beneficial, try doing your deep breathing while doing slow breaststroke.

STITCHES See Herbs – herbal bath; Homoeopathy – calendula tincture; Perineal Tears or Episiotomy – Chapter 10.

STRETCH MARKS

These are less likely if you exercise during your pregnancy and massage your body regularly with a good vegetable oil (see Useful Addresses).

THRUSH

Live yoghurt is very soothing and can help to get rid of thrush (apply locally). If yoghurt doesn't help, try douching with a warm solution of bicarbonate of soda. Consult a homoeopath.

TWINS

If you are carrying twins the yoga-based exercises in this book are especially useful. In late pregnancy be sure to have plenty of rest and follow the cautionary notes carefully when reading the exercise instructions. Sometimes twins are born prematurely, so it is important to give birth in a hospital which has intensive care facilities for newborns. If there are no complications and both babies are a good size there is a good possibility of an active birth. As twins tend to be smaller than singletons, birth may in fact be easier. The position that the babies are lying in during labour can affect the outcome. Both babies may be head down and this is the best outlook for twins. However, often the second twin presents in the breech position. If this is the case an active birth is possible with careful vigilance on the part of the attendants. If there is a problem obstetric intervention will be used. Sometimes the second twin lies sideways (transverse) and can be turned head down manually from the outside before birth.

After the birth of the first twin bonding can take place as usual as first contact between mother and baby will stimulate the contractions which will expel the second twin. The cord need not be cut or clamped immediately. The second twin will probably be born soon after the first and both placentas will be expelled at the end in the usual way.

The supported standing squat (see p 118) is the best position to use for a twin birth. As the placental site is larger with twins, there may be more bleeding than is usual with singletons.

It is a good idea to make contact with a breastfeeding counsellor (see Useful Addresses) before the babies are born to get useful suggestions about breastfeeding twins. Contact with other parents of twins will be helpful. Try to arrange plenty of help at home in the first few weeks.

URINATING

In labour: once every hour.

After labour: this can sting if you have a graze or have torn or had an episiotomy. It helps to use a bowl of warm water with some calendula tincture in it or to pour a jug of warm water between your legs into the toilet as you urinate.

See Herbal bath.

VARICOSE VEINS

The exercise (sequence II, no. 4), 'legs apart on the wall', is helpful as it will aid the return of blood to the upper body. Practise twice daily for 10 minutes. Do only easy squatting using a stool. Put your feet up whenever you get a chance. All the exercises recommended in this book are helpful and will improve your circulation. Comfrey ointment is said to be helpful when applied locally. Avoid standing for long periods and sit on a stool when doing housework tasks wherever possible. Support stockings or tights are helpful. Avoid any exercise that causes pain.

Active Birth Manifesto

1. In every uninhibited labour there is a marked restlessness: the woman walks, stands, squats, kneels, lies down, and moves her body freely to find the most comfortable and appropriate positions. There can be no fixed position for a natural healthy labour and birth when a woman follows her own instincts – for birth is active, involving a succession of changing positions, and is not a passive 'confinement'.
2. Figures reveal that throughout the world today, for the most part, women still labour and deliver in some form of upright or crouching position – usually supported. Whatever the race or tribe: African, American, Asian, and so on, the same upright positions always predominate. For primitive women they are spontaneous and natural. Historians entirely confirm the evidence of the ethnologists showing the prevalent use of vertical positions through the ages.
3. Most women in the western world are confined in hospital in a recumbent position. This practice is illogical and unnecessary. Because of this blind spot, birth in our modern hospitals becomes daily more complicated and expensive, turning a perfectly natural process into a medical event and the labouring woman into a passive patient. No other species adopts such a disadvantageous posture at such a crucial time.
4. Research reveals serious disadvantages to the recumbent posture in labour:
- Lying on one's back is the only position that causes compression of the major abdominal vessels along the spinal column; compression of the large artery of the heart (descending aorta) can cause foetal distress by hindering circulation to the uterus and placenta. Compression of the large veins leading to the heart (inferior vena cava) blocks the returning blood flow contributing to hypotension and other circulatory problems.
- The recumbent position does not take advantage of the mobility of the pelvic muscles. It ignores the help of flexing the knees and hips, i.e. the acute angle made by bringing the knees towards the chest (as in squatting) which opens and widens the pelvis to its maximum. In the reclining position the weight of the body on the sacrum closes the pelvic outlet to its maximum, losing approximately 30 per cent of the possible opening compared to squatting.
- When lying back without any trunk flexion the direction of the uterus's force defies gravity. It is easier for any object to fall towards the earth's surface than to slide parallel to it (Newton's law of gravity). It is more advantageous to expel an unborn baby towards the earth than to expel it along the horizon, which wastes energy and effort, causes unnecessary pain and increases the duration of labour.
- When lying down for delivery the perineal tissues stretch unevenly at the expense of the posterior part, this increases the risk of perineal tearing and the need for episiotomy and certainly increases stress and pain.
5. Position change is more important than a single optimal or best position during labour. However, squatting is the position closest to nature's laws and is known as the physiological position. A birth position is physiologically effective:
- when there is no compression on the blood vessels
- when the pelvis becomes fully mobilized
- when the body works in harmony with the force of gravity

Supported squatting is especially efficient at the end of delivery. The squatting position produces:

- maximum pressure inside the pelvis
- minimal muscular effort
- optimal relaxation of the perineum
- optimal foetal oxygenation.

In the squatting position the entrance of the baby's head or presenting part to the mother's pelvic inlet is easier, and the head's direct application to the mother's cervix is assisted, because the pelvic inlet points forward and the outlet downward producing a convenient angle for descent.

6.   We believe – as numerous studies in the last 50 years indicate – that when birth is active the advantages are:

- the natural rhythm and continuity of birth are not disrupted
- uterine contractions are stronger, more regular and more frequent
- the dilation or opening of the cervix (neck of the womb) is enhanced
- more complete relaxation is possible between contractions while interuterine pressure is consistently higher
- the first and second stages of labour are shorter

Some comparative studies showed over 40 per cent shorter time in the upright group.

- there is greater comfort, less stress and pain and so decreased requirement for analgesia
- improved condition of the newborn
- women feel they are fully participating, and in control of their labours and more often experience giving birth as a wonderful and joyous experience.

7.   After an active birth, the mother feels that she has given birth rather than having had her baby extracted from her. She and her baby have been full participants together and are both alert, undrugged and healthy when they meet face to face. This inevitably results in the best possible parent-child bonding.

8.   As well as celebration in the family, the birth of every child is a critical, uncertain event, involving suspense as to the final outcome. The skill of giving birth and the skill of birth attendants is prized by every society. We believe that in the modern western world, through technology, the skill of the attendants has completely over-balanced the skill of the giver of birth, so that most women have lost the knack of giving birth skillfully.

Childbirth, in any woman's life, is an exceptional act, a *tour de force*, partly instinct and partly knack. There is a knack to doing most things and giving birth is no exception. We believe that this balance of skill and power must be restored by increasing the skill and power of the giver of birth, the mother.

9.   Based on research findings, various up to date studies, and ancestral instinct, it is foreseeable that certain changes in respect to labour and birth positions are inevitable in the management of labour and in the preparation of women for childbirth. A prospective mother needs not merely knowledge of pregnancy, labour and delivery, the growth and development of babies, but also adequate physical preparation. She needs to know the effects of varying upright positions and to cultivate ease and comfort in them to enable her to actively and effectively help herself when giving birth to her children.

She can also benefit greatly from learning to quieten her mind and become more deeply in touch with her inner self and her deep instinctive potential for giving birth.

10.   Finally, there is no doubt to any woman who has experienced an active birth herself, or to anyone who has witnessed many active and passive births, that an active labour and birth is easier, safer and more rewarding for both mother and child. The way our children are born affects their lives and any improvement in the birth experience helps us towards a better world. Usually a natural birth merely refers to a labour where no pharmaceutical drugs have been used, whereas an active birth is, in the full sense of the phrase, a truly natural birth.

Written by J. and A. Balaskas, 1982

References for the Active Birth Manifesto

Caldeyro-Barcia, R., 'The influence of maternal position on time of spontaneous rupture of the membranes, progress of labour, and foetal head compression', Birth and Fam. J. 6 : 7, 1979.

Noriega-Gerra, L., Cibils, L. A., Alvarez, H., Proseiro, J. J., Pose, S. V., Sica-Blanco, Y., Mendez-Bauer, C., Fielita, C., Gonzales-Panizzva, V. H., 'Effect of position changes on the intensity and frequency of uterine contractions during labour', Am. J. Obstet. Gynecol. 80 : 284–290, 1960; 'Supine called worst position during labour and delivery', Ob. Gyn. News June: 1 & 54, 1975.

Chan, D., 'Positions in labour', Br. Med. J. 5323 : 100–102, 1963.

Clarke, A. P., 'The influence of position of the patient in labour in causing uterine inertia and pelvic disturbances', JAMA 16 : 433–435, 1891.

Diaz, A. G., Schqarez, R., Fescina y, R., Caldeyro-Barcia, R., 'Efectos de la posicion vertical materna sobre la evolution del parto', Separata de la Revista Clinica e Investigacion en Ginecologia y Obstetricia 3 : 101–109, 1978.

Dunn, P., 'Posture in labour', Lancet 1, 8062 : 496–497, 1978.

Flynn, A. M., Kelly, J., Hollins, G., Lynch, P. F., 'Ambulation in labour', Br. Med. J. 2 : 591–593, 1978.

Flynn, A., Kelly, J., 'Continuous foetal monitoring in the ambulant patient in labour', Br. Med. J. 2 : 842–843, 1976.

Hugo, M., 'A look at maternal position during labour', J. Nurs-Midwif 22 : 26–27, 1977.

Humphrey, M., Hunslow, D., Morgan, S., Wood, C., 'The influence of maternal posture at birth on the foetus', J. Obstet. Gynaecol. Brit. Commonw. 80 : 1075–1080, 1973.

Kouvenen, K., Teramo, K., 'Effect of maternal position on fetal heart during extradural analgesia', Br. J. Anaesth. 51 : 767, 1979.

King, A. F. A., 'The significance of posture in obstetrics', NY Med. J. 80 : 1054–1058, 1909.

Liu, Y. C., 'Effects of an upright position during labour', Am. J. Nurs. 74 : 2202–2205, 1974. 'Position during labour and delivery: history and perspective', J. Nurs-Midwif 24 : 23–26, 1979.

Mendez-Bauer, C., Arroyo, J., Carciaramos, C., Menendez, A., Lavilla, M., Lzquierdo, F., Elizaga, I. V., Zamarriego, J., 'Effects of standing position on spontaneous uterine contractility and other aspects of labour', J. Perinat Med. 3 : 89–100, 1975.

Arroyo, J., Menendez, A., Salmean, J., Manas, J., Lavilla, M., Martin, S. M., Elizaga, I. V., Crespo, J. Z., 'Effects of different positions during labour', Fifth European Congress of Perinatal Medicine, Sweden, 1976.

Mendez-Bauer, C., Arroyo, J., Zamarriego, J., 'Maternal standing position in first stage of labour', 'Reviews in Perinatal Medicine' Vol. 1, Edited by E. M. Scarpelli and E. V. Cosmi, Baltimore, University Park Press, 1976, pp. 281–293.

Arroyo, J., Reina, A., Menendez, S., Zamarriego, J. O., *Monitoring and Maternal Posture, Sixth European Congress of Perinatal Medicine*, Edited by O. Thalhammer, K. Baungarten and A. Pollak, Stuttgart, Georg Thieme, 1979, pp. 294–295.

McKay, S., 'Maternal position during labour and birth', ICEA Rev. 2 : 3, 1978.

Markoe, J. W., 'Posture in obstetrics', Bulletin Lying-in-Hosp. NY 11 : 11–26, 1917.

Mitre, I. N., 'The influence of maternal position on duration of the active phase of labour', Int. J. Gynaecol. Obstet. 12 : 181–183, 1974.

McManus, T. J., Calder, A. A., 'Upright posture and the efficiency of labour', Lancet i. 8055 : 72–74, 1978.

Roberts, J. E., 'Maternal positions for childbirth – an historical review of nursing care practices', J. Obstet. Gynecol. Neo. Nurs. 8(1) : 24–32, 1979.

Manion, C. V., 'Posture in labour', Lancet 1, 8062 : 497, 1978.

Roberts, J. 'Alternative frontiers for childbirth', J. of Nurse Midwifery. July/Aug. 1980. Vol. 25, n. 4.

Rhodes, P., 'Posture in obstetrics', Physiotherapy 53 : 158–163, 1967.

Scambler, A., 'Stand and deliver', Mims. Mag. 15.6.80.

Williams, R. M., Thom, M. H., Studd, J. W. W., 'A study of the benefits and acceptability of ambulation in spontaneous labour', Brit. J. obst. & gynol. Feb. 1980. Vol. 87.

Odent, Michel, *Bien-naitre, Genèse de l'homme ecologique.*

Recommended Reading

Exercise
Balaskas, J. and A., *New Life: The Exercise Book for Childbirth* (Sidgwick & Jackson 1983)
Tobias, Maxine and Stewart, Mary, *Stretch and Relax* (Dorling Kindersley 1985)
Hoare, Sophy, *Yoga and Pregnancy* (Unwin Paperbacks 1985)
Dale, Barbara and Roeber, Johanna, *Exercise for Childbirth* (Century 1982)
Noble, Elizabeth, *Essential Exercises for the Childbearing Year* (John Murray 1980)
Whiteford, Barbara and Polden, Maggie, *Postnatal Exercises* (Century 1984)

Pregnancy and birth
Balaskas, Janet and Gordon, Yehudi, *The Encyclopaedia of Pregnancy and Birth* (Macdonald Orbis 1987)
Odent, Michel, *Primal Health* (Century 1986)
Kitzinger, Sheila, *Pregnancy and Childbirth* (Michael Joseph 1980)
Odent, Michel, *Birth Reborn* (Fontana 1986)
Junor, Vikki and Monaco, Marianne, *Homebirth Handbook* (Souvenir Press 1984)
Kitzinger, Sheila and Davis, John A., *The Place of Birth* (OUP 1978)
Sidenbladh, Erik, *Water Babies* (Adam & Charles Black 1983)

Fathers
Balaskas, Janet, *The Active Birth Partner's Handbook* (Sidgwick & Jackson 1984)
Roeber, Johanna, *Shared Parenthood – A Handbook for Fathers* (Century 1987)
Bradman, Tony, *The Essential Father* (Unwin Paperbacks 1985)

Midwifery
Flint, Caroline, *Sensitive Midwifery* (Heinemann 1986)
Gaskin, Ina May, *Spiritual Midwifery* (The Book Publishing Co., USA 1977)
Davis, Elizabeth, *Guide to Midwifery – Heart and Hands* (John Muir Publications, USA)

Parents' rights
Beech, Beverley, *Who's Having your Baby? – A Health Rights Handbook to Maternity Care* (Camden Press 1987)
Inch, Sally, *Birth Rights* (Hutchinson 1982)
Stanway, Andrew and Penny, *Choices in Childbirth* (Pan 1984)
Kitzinger, Sheila, *Freedom and Choice in Childbirth* (Penguin 1988)
Haire, Doris, 'The Cultural Warping of Childbirth', *Childbirth Educator*, Spring 1987 (available from ICEA)
Haire, Doris, 'How the FDA determines the "safety" of drugs – just how safe is "safe"?', a report to United States Congress, National Women's Health Network (available from ICEA)

Parenting
Walker, Peter and Fiona, *Natural Parenting* (Bloomsbury 1987)
Walker, Peter, *Baby Relax* (Unwin Paperbacks 1986)
Walker, Peter, *Baby Massage* (Bloomsbury 1988)
Laing, R. D., *The Facts of Life* (Penguin 1977)
Winnicott, D. W., *The Child, the Family and the Outside World* (Penguin 1969)
Kennell, John and Klaus, Marshall, *Maternal Infant Bonding* (USA)
Pearce, Joseph Chiltern, *Magical Child* (Granada)
Kitzinger, Sheila, *Women as Mothers* (Fontana 1978)
Thevenin, Tine, *The Family Bed – An age old concept in child rearing*
Liedloff, Jean, *The Continuum Concept* (Futura 1976)

Breastfeeding

Kitzinger, Sheila, *The Experience of Breastfeeding* (Penguin 1979)

La Leche League International, *The Womanly Art of Breastfeeding* (Souvenir Press 1970, Tandem 1975)

Gaskin, Ina May, *Babies, Breastfeeding and Bonding* (Bergin & Ganvey Publishing USA)

Stanway, Andrew and Penny, *Breast is Best* (Pan 1978)

Messenger, Maire, *The Breastfeeding Book* (Century 1982)

Water Birth

Sidenbladh, Erik, *Water Babies* (Adam & Charles Black 1983)

Daniels, Karil, *The Water Baby Information Book* (Point of View Productions USA)

Massage

Lidell, Lucinda, *The Book of Massage* (Ebury press)

Thomas, Sara, *Massage for Common Ailments* (Collins)

Video on Active Birth by Janet Balaskas.

Yoga for Active Birth (audio cassette), available from the Active Birth Centre.

Useful Addresses

The Active Birth Movement
55 Dartmouth Park Road, London NW5 1SL. Telephone 01-267-3006
Aids and Pregnancy: Healthline (confidential telephone information service)
Telephone 01-980-4848 (6–10pm)
Association for the Improvement in Maternity Services (AIMS)
163 Liverpool Road, London N1
Association of Radical Midwives (ARM)
62 Greetby Hill, Ormskirk, Lancashire L39 2DT
British Acupuncture Association and Register
34 Alderney Street, London SW1V 4EU
British Homoeopathic Association
27a Devonshire Street, London W1
Independent Midwives Association
65 Mount Nod Road, Streatham, London SW16 2LP
International Childbirth Education Association (ICEA)
PO Box 20048, Minneapolis, MN 55420-0048, USA
La Leche League
BCM 3424, London WC1N 3XX
Meet-a-Mum Association (MAMA)
c/o Valerie Dallinger, 5 Westbury Avenue, Luton, Beds LU2 7DW
National Childbirth Trust
Alexandra House, Oldham Terrace, Acton, London W3 6NH
National Council for One-Parent Families
255 Kentish Town Road, London NW5 2LX
National Institute of Medical Herbalists
Secretary: Janet Hicks, 41 Hatherly Road, Winchester, Hants

Osteopathy Pregnancy Clinic
The British School of Osteopathy, Littlejohn House, 1–4 Suffolk Street, London SW1
Patients Association
18 Victoria Park Square, Bethnall Green, London E2 9PF
Royal College of Midwives
15 Mansfield Street, London W1
Society of Homoeopaths
101, Sebastian Avenue, Shenfield, Brentwood, Essex CM15 8PP
Society to Support Home Confinements
17 Laburnum Avenue, Durham

Beauty Birth
144 Campden High Street, London NW1 0NE
(a mail order list of pure oils especially prepared for pregnancy and labour)
Homoeopathic remedies can be obtained from some chemists and health food stores or a homoeopathic pharmacy such as A. Nelson & Co., 73 Duke Street, London W1 or by post from 5 Endeavour Way, Wimbledon, London SW19 9UH; or Ainsworths Homoeopathic Pharmacy, 38 New Cavendish Street, London W1.
Yoga mats may be bought from R & J White, Church Farm House, Spring Close Lane, Cheam, Surrey SM3 8PU.
Water birth pools from The Active Birth Centre, 55 Dartmouth Park Road, London NW5.

Australia
Parents' Centres Australia
c/o Andrea Robertson, PO Box 398, Parramatta, NSW
La Leche League Australia
c/o Pinky McKay, 8 Gateshead Drive, Wantirna, Vic 3152
Childbirth Education Association
PO Box 413, Hurstville, NSW 2220
Homebirth Access
PO Box 66, Broadway, NSW 2007
Nursing Mothers Association of Australia
PO Box 231, Nunawading, Vic 3131
Dial-a-mum Association of Australia
PO Box 241, Wahroonga, NSW 2076
Maternity Alliance
PO Box 107, Lawson, NSW 2783
Associates in Childbirth Education
148 Hereford Street, Forest Lodge, NSW 2037

New Zealand
Childbirth Education Network
Pauline Scott, PO Box 7042, Tauranga
Plunket Society
3 Moncrief Street, Mount Victoria, Wellington
La Leche League New Zealand
Box 13 383, Wellington 4
New Zealand Parents' Centres
PO Box 11310, Wellington.

Reference List

Chapter 1

1. Prentice, 'Foetal heartrate monitoring during labour – too frequent intervention, too little benefit?' *Lancet*, Vol. 2 No. 8572, December 1987, pages 1375–1377.
2. National statistic for 1986 (USA).
3. Doris Haire is a medical sociologist. She is President of the American Foundation for Maternal and Child Health, Founder of CEA, former President of ICEA and former Chair of the National Women's Health Network USA (see Recommended Reading, Useful Addresses).
4. Haire, Doris, 'Drugs in Labour' *Childbirth Educator* Spring 1987 (USA).
5. Bowes, W., *et al.*, 'The side effects of obstetrical medication on fetus and infant' Monographs of the Society for Research in Child Development, No. 137 Vol. 35, June 1970.
   Brazelton, T. B., 'Effect of maternal medications on the neonate and his behaviour' *Journal of Pediatrics* (USA) 58 : 513–518, 1961.
   Rosenblatt, D., 'The influence of maternal analgesia on neonatal behaviour' *British Journal of Obstetrics and Gynaecology* Vol. 88, April 1981, pages 398–406.
   Kron, R., 'Newborn sucking behaviour affected by obstetric sedation' *Pediatrics* (USA) 37 : 1012–1016, 1966.
6. Rosenblatt, D., 'The influence of maternal analgesia on neonatal behaviour' *British Journal of Obstetrics and Gynaecology*, Vol. 88, April 1986, pages 398–406.
7. Maclerian and Carrie, *British Medical Journal* January 1977, pages 14–16.
8. Hubinot, P. *et al.*, 'Effects of vacuum extractor and obstetrical forceps on the foetus and newborn – a comparison' World Congress on Gynaecology and Obstetrics, Sydney, Australia, 1967.
9. Rosenblatt, D., 'Epidural Buvacaine' *British Journal of Obstetrics and Gynaecology* Vol. 88, April 1981, pages 407–417.
10. Johnson, W., 'Regionals can prolong labour' *Medical World News* October 1971.
11. Potter, N. and Macdonald, R., 'Obstetric consequences of epidural analgesia on nulliparous patients' *Lancet* 1 : 1031–1034, May 1971.
12. Hellman, L. and Pritchard, J., *Williams Obstetrics* 14th ed. (Appleton, Century-Crofts, NY 1971).
13. Taylor, R. W., 'Misuse of oxytocin in labour' Letter to *Lancet*, February 1988.
14. Chalmers, I., Campbell, H. and Turnbull, A., 'Use of oxytocin and incidence of neonatal jaundice' *British Medical Journal* 2 : 116.
15. Steer, P. *et al.*, *British Journal of Obstetrics and Gynaecology* Vol. 92, November 1985, pages 1120–1126.
16. Fields, H., 'Induction of labour: Methods, hazards, complications and contraindications' *Hospital Topics* December 1968, pages 63–68.
17. Fields, H., 'Complications of elective induction' *Obstetrics and Gynaecology* 15 : 476–480, 1960.
18. Liston and Campbell, 'Dangers of oxytocin induced labour to the fetus' *British Medical Journal* 1974.
19. Russell, J. G. B., 'Moulding of the pelvic outlet' *British Journal of Obstetric and Gynaecology* Commonwealth 76, 1969, pages 817–820.
20. Scott, D. B. and Kerr, M. G., 'Interior vena canal pressure in late pregnancy' *Journal of Obstetrics and Gynaecology* British Commonwealth Volume 70, page 1044–1963.
21. Flynn, A. M., Kelly, J., Hollins, G. and Lynch, P. F., 'Ambulation in labour' *British Medical Journal* August 1978, pages 591–593.
22. Caldeyro-Barcia, R., 'The influence of maternal position on time of spontaneous rupture of the membranes, progress of labour and foetal head compression' *Birth and Family* J6 : 7 1979.
23. Mitie, I. N., 'The influence of maternal position on duration of the active phase of labour' *International Journal of Gynaecology and Obstetrics* 12, 1974, pages 181–183.
24. Lui, Y. C., 'Effects of an upright position during labour' *American Journal of Nursing* 74, 1974, pages 2202–2205.
   Lui, Y. C., 'Position during labour and delivery : history and perspective' *J. Nurse-Midwife* 24 : 1979, pages 23–26.

25. Dunn, P., *Lancet* 1, 8062 : pages 492–497, 1978.
26. Botha, M., 'The management of the umbilical cord in labour' *South African Journal of Obstetrics* 6(2) : 30–33, 1968.
27. Blankfield, A., 'The optimum position for childbirth' *Medical Journal Australia* 2 : 1965, pages 666–668.
28. Howard, F. H., 'Delivery in the physiologic position' *Obstetrics and Gynaecology* 11 : 1958, pages 318–322.
29. Gritsivk, I., 'Position in labour' *Obstetrics-Gynaecology Observer* September 1968.
30. Newton, N., and Newton, M., 'The propped position for the second stage of labour' *Obstetrics and Gynaecology* 15 : 1960, pages 28–34.

Chapter 6
1. Odent, Michel, 'The Fetus Ejection Reflex' *Birth* (USA) 14 : June 1987.
   Newton, N., 'The Fetus Ejection Reflex Revisited' *Birth* (USA) 14 : June 1987.
2. Newton, N., Foshee, D. and Newton, M., 'Experimental inhibition of labour through environmental disturbance' *Obstetrics and Gynaecology* 1966, 67, pages 371–377.

Chapter 7
1. Photographs as well as information about Igor Tjarkovsky and his work can be obtained from *Water Babies* by Erik Sidenbladh (Adam & Charles Black 1983).
2. see reference no. 6 for Chapter 7.
3. Sidenbladh, E., *Water Babies*, page 58.
4. Odent, Michel, 'Birth under Water' *Lancet*, December 24/31 1983.
5. Odent, Michel, *Birth Reborn*.
6. International contacts for Water Birth and a video entitled 'Water Baby – Experiences of Water Birth' can be obtained from the *Water Baby Information Book* by Karil Daniels (Point of View Productions, 2477 Folsom Street, San Fransisco, LA 94110, USA).
7. Rosenthal, M., 'Water Birth: An American Experience' in the *Water Birth Information Book* by Karil Daniels.
8. Tjarkovsky maintains that this is unlikely to increase the risk of infection as you share the same bacteriological environment as your partner.
9. For local contacts or further details about the dimensions, hire or purchase of water pools contact the Active Birth Centre (see Useful Addresses).

Index

Note: bold figures denote illustrations or photographs

abdominal cavity **18**
abdominal toner 66–7, **67**
accelerating labour 174–5
active birth 1
  advantages of 11–13
  at home or in hospital 161–90
  implications of 13–14
  and obstetrics 182–4
Active Birth Movement ix–x
  Manifesto 201–2
alcohol 191
all-fours position
  tuck-ins exercise 50, **50**
  in second stage 131–2, **131–3**
anaemia 191
ankle release exercise 41
anterior lip, knee-chest position for 110, **111**
anterior position 176
artificial rupture of membranes (Arm/amniotomy) 191–2
awareness of baby and meditation 39

baby
  bathing of 125, **127**
  and breastfeeding 150–4, **152–3**
  crowning of head 114–15, **119**
  during second stage 111–13, **112, 119–23**
  during transition **109**, 110
  immediately after birth 134–5
  monitoring for active birth 171–3
  unusual presentations 175–9, **176–7, 179**
  in womb at term 94–5, **95–6**
  see also birth

backache 192
back massage 86–7, **86–7**
basic sitting exercise (yoga) 36, **37**
birth attendants 188
birth
  active *see* active birth
  after *see* postnatal period; third stage of labour
  before obstetrics 7–8
  induction to ease 6–7
  labour and 88–138, **119–23**
  water *see* water birth
birth room (at home) 164–5, 189–90
birthstool 8
bleeding 192
blood pressure 192–3
breast(s) 193
  care 153
breastfeeding 193
  how it works 151–3, **152–3**
  in later months 154
  starting 150–1
breathing 79–82
  exercise (yoga) 38–9
  during labour 81–2
  for first stage of labour 99
  for second stage 115–16
  for transition 111
  what happens when we breathe 79–81, **80**
breech presentation 162, 176–8, **177, 179**
bupivacaine 186

Caesarian births 3, 6, 7
Caldeyro-Barcia, Dr Roberto 10
calf
  massage 88
  stretch exercise 60, **60**

cervix
  dilation **109**
  and labour 94–7, **95–6**, 108, **109**
constipation 193
contractions
  first-stage labour 95–100, **95, 98**
cramp 193
crowning 114–15

deep pressure (massage) 83
deep stroking 82
Demerol (US) *see* Pethidine
dog pose exercise 61–3, **61–2**
drugs *see* medication
due date 193–4
Dunn, Dr Peter 11

eating in labour 194
emergency birth 194–5
Englemann, Dr G. J. *Labour Among
    Primitive Peoples* 9
Entenox (gas and oxygen) 186
epidurals 5–6, 183
episiotomy 181–2
exercises *see* postnatal exercises; yoga-based
    exercises during pregnancy; *see also
    specific exercises*

first stage of labour 94–107, **95–6, 98,
    100–7**
  using water during 141–3, **142**
fluid retention (oedema) 195
foetal distress 195–6
foot massage 88
forceps delivery 2, 3, 6, 183–4
forward bend exercise 56, **57**

gas and oxygen (Entenox) 186

haemorrhoids (piles) 196
Haire, Doris 6
  Cultural Warping of Childbirth, The 4
  Drugs in Labour and Birth 6
half-kneeling, half-squatting 106, **107**
  in second stage (side lying) 133–4, **134**
head
  and neck massage 85
  roll exercise 52, **53**
headaches 196

heart and lungs during pregnancy 29
heartburn 196
herbs 196–7
home, active birth at 160–5, 197
homoeopathy 197–8
hospital, active birth in 160–3, 165–71
  movements for labour 167–9, **168–9**
  what to take with you 166–7

induction 6–7, 187, 198
insomnia 198
internal examination 173–4

jaundice 198

kneading 84
knee bend exercise 42, **42**
knee-chest position for anterior lip 110, **111**
kneeling
  in second stage (all-fours position)
    131–2, **131–3**
  exercises 45–50, **45–51**
  position in labour **104–7**, 105–6, **169**

labour x, 1, 88–138
  accelerating 174–5
  eating in 194
  exercise for 50, **51**
  inducing 6–7, 187, 198
  sensations of 91–2
  suggestions for 17
  see also first stage; second stage; third
    stage; transition
leaning forward in labour 103, **103, 168**
Leboyer, Frederick 140
leg exercises
  apart on the wall 68–71, **68**
  wide apart 42, **43**
lower back release exercise 74–5, **75**

massage 83–8
  for pregnancy 84–8, **86–7**
maternal organs **19**
Mauriceau, François 8
medication and active birth 184–7
meditation and baby awareness 39
midwife
  and delivery 124–5
  examination by **101**

miscarriage 199
Mitie, Dr Isaac N. 10
monitoring baby for active birth 171–3
morning sickness 199

obstetrics
    active birth and 182–4
    birth before 7–8
    drawbacks of births managed by 4–5
Odent, Michel 15–16, **140**, 140–3
oedema (fluid retention) 195
orgasm 199
oxytocin or syntocin drip 187

pain in delivery 92–4
    drugs for 5–6
paracervical block 187
pelvic bones and joints 22–8, **22–8**
    muscles attached to **28**
pelvic floor 26–7, **27**
    exercises 65–6, **65**
        postnatal 156–60, **156**
pelvic lift 49, **49**
    for spinal release and relaxation 72–3, **73**
pelvic organs 18–22, **18**
pelvic release exercise 39–44
perineal tears 180–1
    how to avoid 180
    repairing 181
pethidine (Demerol in USA) 5, 185
piles (haemorrhoids) 196
Pithiviers, France, maternity in 15–16
    use of water 140
placenta
    praevia 163
    separation of **123**, 135–8, **136–7**
placental insufficiency 199
positions
    for delivery 2
    ethnological evidence 9
    in first stage 99–107, **100–7**
    recent studies 9–10
    results of modern research 10–11
    in second stage 116–35, **118–20, 122,
        124, 126, 128–34**
    in transition 110
    in underwater birth 144
posterior presentation 175–6, **176**

postnatal period 149–54
    breast care 153
    breastfeeding 150–4
    exercises during 155–60, **156–9**
    your body during 149–50
    see also third stage of labour
pre-eclampsia or toxaemia 162
pregnancy
    sun salute exercise 53–6, **54–5**
    your body in 18–29
presentations
    breech 162, 176–8, **177, 179**
    posterior 175–6, **176**
    transverse 178–9
    unusual 175–9

reclining positions 66–71, **67–8, 70–1**
    exercises with partner 69–70, **70–1**
    for spinal release and relaxation 72, **72**
relaxation exercises 78, **78**
    postnatal 157, **157**
resting in between contractions 105–6, **105**
rhesus factor 199–200

sacro-illiac joints 25–6, **25–6**
second stage of labour 111–35, **112,
        118–24, 126–34**
    in hospital 169–71
self-massage 84–5
shoulder stand exercise 158–60, **159**
side lying 133–4, **134**
sitting position in labour 103, **103, 169**
slowing down labour 110, **111**, 175
spinal release and relaxation 72–8, **72–8**
spinal twist exercises 47–8, **48**, 75, **76**
    with partner 76–7, **77**
spine during pregnancy 28–9, **29**
sport 200
squatting 14–15
    exercises 60–6, **60–2, 64–5**
    in labour 102–3, **102, 170–1**
    supported *see* supported squatting
    in water birth pool 141–2, **142**
standing positions 51–7, **51–5, 57**
    in labour 99–100, **100**
stillbirth 187–8
stomach massage 88
stretch marks 200

supported squatting 118–31, **118–24, 169–71**
  with two people 127–30, **129–30**
  using a chair 130–1, **130**
surface and deep stroking 83
syntocin or oxytocin in drip 187

tailor pose 39–40, **40**
  advanced posture 41, **41**
tears, avoiding and repairing 181–2
thigh massage 88
third stage of labour 135–8, **136–7**
  and water birth 145–6
  see also postnatal period
thrush 200
Tjarkovsky, Igor 139
toxaemia or pre-eclampsia 162
transition stage (end of labour) 108–11, **109, 111**
trilene 187
twins 200

underwater birth *see* water birth
unusual presentations 175–9, **176–7, 179**
urinating 200
uterus 18–22, **18–20**, 27, **27**
  contractions 97, **98**

valium 185
varicose veins 201
ventouse 183–4

warm up, for standing postures 52
water birth 139–48
  after the birth 147
  giving birth under water 143–5
  history 139–41
  positions for 144
  practicalities 147–8
  preparing for 148
  third stage 145–6
  using water during first stage 141–3
Western practice, modern 2–4

yoga-based exercises during pregnancy 30–78
  benefits of 33–4
  breathing 38–9
  getting centred 36–9
  how yoga works 31–2
  meditation and basic awareness 39
  useful tips 36
  warning 35–6
  and water birth 148
  see also specific exercises
Yuen Chou Lui, Dr 10